Atlas of Anatomy of the Hand

Atlas of Anatomy of the Hand

JOHAN M. F. LANDSMEER

Professor of Anatomy and Embryology
University of Leiden

CHURCHILL LIVINGSTONE Edinburgh London and New York 1976

CHURCHILL LIVINGSTONE

Medical Division of Longman Group Limited

Distributed in the United States of America by
Longman Inc., 19 West 44th Street, New York,
N.Y. 10036 and associated companies,
branches and representatives throughout the world.

ISBN 0 443 01154 0

Library of Congress Catalog Card Number 74—82392

First edition 1976
  Reprinted 1977

Printed in Great Britain by
William Clowes & Sons, Limited
London, Beccles and Colchester

To my wife
Annelies

and my children
Arie
Meindert
Jasper
Janneke

Preface

Because of its spatial and pictorial aspects, morphology has always posed particular problems of storage and transmission of knowledge. Being aware of these problems and of the strong demand for detailed structural information, I felt that there was a need for an analysis of the hand in serial sections, whereby structural and spatial relationships are kept intact. This book, I hope, fulfils the need. It is intended primarily as a reference source of old and new information on the hand and as a guide to surgical approaches and anatomical explorations.

The book is thus designed for both anatomists and surgeons, for both trainees and teachers. It provides a comprehensive anatomical basis for the growing number of postgraduates specializing in hand surgery.

The book has been divided into nine chapters, the first offering a general survey of the subject. Each chapter is designed as an independent unit, complete in itself, so that inevitably some overlap exists between them. Structure and function are virtually inseparable in practice, and it is hoped that by the inclusion of a chapter on functional aspects, the scope of the book is widened.

In view of the structure of the book, a detailed table of contents has been provided instead of an index, in the belief that the former will prove much more helpful to the reader. The figure legends have been made as informative as possible. The large number of illustrations should provide opportunity for the reader to check the analysis presented against his own observations.

References to the relevant literature are made in the general discussion. Kaplan's bibliography gives unparalleled access to sources as far back as Albinus, Weitbrecht and Camper. All involved in research on the hand are indebted to Stack, not only for an extensive bibliography on the palmar fascia, but also for the reproduction of the related classical texts, either translated or in the original. My intention in designing this book has been to present the available literature and to provide a structural analytical plan permitting critical assessment of data extracted from the literature or derived from one's own observations.

The investigations on which this book is based were carried out in the Department of Anatomy and Embryology at Leiden. This work would not have been possible without the co-operation and the incomparable craftsmanship of illustrators, photographers and technicians. Directly concerned with the book were Jan Tinkelenberg and later also Henk Wetselaar, who produced the illustrations, and Hans Bles, who saw to the photographic documentation.

The writer would like to mention the most able assistance of Annelies Oosterling-Wolkers during the first years of the work and Jeannette de Jong during completion of the manuscript and correction of the proofs. Heartfelt thanks and admiration go to Dr Ruby May Collister for the correction of the English text. Finally the writer acknowledges gratefully the work undertaken by Churchill Livingstone in making available in print this extensive documentary material. Their applied expertise, the care and devotion given to text and illustrations, have given the author a deep sense of satisfaction.

Leiden   Johan M. F. Landsmeer

Acknowledgements

The author is grateful to the editors of the journals specified below and to certain of his colleagues for permission to reproduce the following illustrations:

Figure 9.1
Acta anatomica (1968) Suppl. 54, **70,** Fig. 33, p. 65. Published by S. Karger AG, Basel.

Figure 9.2
Acta Morphologica Neerlando-Scandinavica (1960) **3,** No. 3–4, Fig. 18f, p. 314.

Figure 9.3
Annals of Rheumatic Diseases (1962) **21,** No. 2, Fig. 2a, p. 167. Published by the British Medical Association, London.

Figure 9.4b
Acta anatomica (1955) Suppl. 24, **25,** Fig. 26, p. 40. Published by S. Karger AG, Basel.

Figure 9.5
Journal of Bone and Joint Surgery (1963) **45-A,** No. 8, Figs. 1b & 1c, p. 1655.

Figure 9.7
Acta anatomica (1955) Suppl. 24, **25,** Fig. 20, p. 32. Published by S. Karger AG, Basel.

Figure 9.8
Journal of Bone and Joint Surgery (1963) **45-A,** No. 8, Fig. 2b, p. 1658.

Figure 9.9
Acta anatomica (1968) Suppl. 54, **70,** Fig. 34, p. 67. Published by S. Karger AG, Basel.

Figure 9.10
Acta anatomica (1955) Suppl. 24, **25,** Fig. 29, p. 52. Published by S. Karger AG, Basel.

Figure 9.11
Journal of Bone and Joint Surgery (1968) **50-B,** Figs. 4 & 5, p. 666.

Figure 9.12
Long, C. (1970) *Normal and Abnormal Motor Control in the Upper
Extremities*. Final Report. Social and Rehabilitation Services. Grant No.
RD-2377-M. Dec. 1966 to April 1970, Fig. 11, p. 16b.

Figure 9.13
Acta anatomica (1955) Suppl. 24, **25,** Figs. 33 & 34, p. 61; Figs. 35 & 36,
p. 62. Published by S. Karger AG, Basel.

Figure 9.14
Acta Orthopaedica Scandinavica (1973) Suppl. 148, Fig. III-10, p. 66;
Fig. III-11, p. 67.

Figure 9.15
Acta Orthopaedica Scandinavica (1973) Suppl. 148, Figs. V-9a & V-9b,
p. 98.

Figure 9.16
Ebskov, B. (1970) De motibus motoribusque pollicis humani. Thesis:
Copenhagen, Denmark, Fig. 45, p. 143.

Figure 9.17
Kauer, J.M.G. (1964) Een analyse van de carpale flexie. Thesis: Leiden,
Holland, Fig. 12, p. 60.

Contents

1. General Survey

On studying a series of sections one easily recognizes the well-known features and structures in the hand and these provide a reference system for our observations on the structural and spatial relationships.

The dominant features of the human hand have been mapped out in a limited number of sections which have been selected according to the most characteristic features at the respective levels.

1. Distal radioulnar level.
2. Proximal carpal level.
3. Capitate head level.
4. Distal carpal level.
5. Carpometacarpal transition zone.
6. Basimetacarpal level.
7. Proximal metacarpal level.
8. Midmetacarpal level.
9. Distal metacarpal level.
10. Metacarpophalangeal transition zone.
11. Proximal phalangeal level.
12. Proximal interphalangeal level.
13. Middle phalanx level.
14. Distal interphalangeal level.
15. Third phalanx level (tuberosity).

1. DISTAL RADIOULNAR LEVEL
(Fig. 1.1)

The extensor tendons lie in osteofibrous sheaths, each with its own typical arrangement. The extensor carpi ulnaris sheath is attached to the ulna. The superficial layer of the deep fascia runs freely over it, with an areolar space intervening. The sheaths of extensor digiti V and the extensor communis (including the extensor indicis proprius) are both fibrous slings attached to the radius being rounded on their ulnar aspects; in contrast the sling of the extensor pollicis longus is rounded on its radial aspect. The extensors carpi radialis longus and brevis are held in a sheath which is round on both aspects. The sheaths of the extensor pollicis brevis and of the abductor pollicis longus are seen attached to the styloid process of the radius. The volar fascias are seen to be rather thin. The radial artery and the flexor carpi radialis lie in a fold of the superficial fascia.

2. PROXIMAL CARPAL LEVEL
(Fig. 1.2)

The scaphoid and lunate bones can just be seen in this section. At its interface with the styloid process of the ulna the sheath of extensor carpi ulnaris can be seen to vary its position by what might be called a rolling movement and thus the tendon can change its position in relation to the ulna. A thick anterior fibrous layer represents the distal continuity of the anterior border of the radius. The triangular ligament forms part of the system. The extensor pollicis longus has just entered the sheath of the radial carpal extensors.

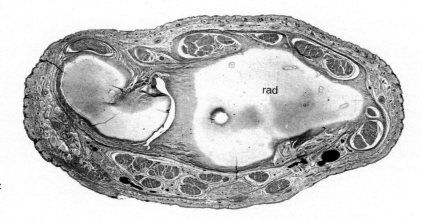

Fig. 1.1 (*series no. 1899*; neg. 15817). Level: 2. Section through the distal radio-ulnar joint. rad=radius.

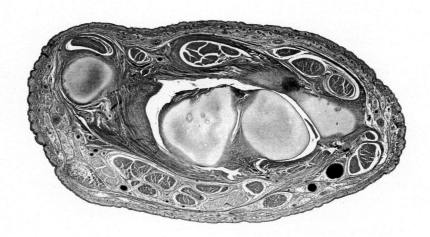

Fig. 1.2 (*series no. 1899*; neg. 15818). Level: 72. Section at proximal carpal level.

3. CAPITATE HEAD LEVEL
(Fig. 1.3.)

The volar ligament layer, which is the distal continuity of the border of the radius and of the triangular ligament, is invaded by the lunate. The flexor carpi ulnaris tendon is already partially replaced by the pisiform bone. Both radial and ulnar bursae have become visible in the flexor compartment and clefts have appeared around the superficial flexor tendons. A marked feature is the indication of the most proximal portion of the hypothenar subcutaneous space (arrow). The head of the capitate forms an extremely well-marked feature at this level, while the difference in the curvatures of its scaphoid and lunate facies cannot be missed. The wedge-shaped sections of the lunate and scaphoid reflect their functional position in the mechanism of the carpus. The sheath of the extensor carpi ulnaris is seen to be more or less isolated from the fibrous continuity of the styloid process; it is firmly fixed, however, to the triquetrum, as are the distal insertion of the triangular ligament, the dorsal radiocarpal ligament and the scaphotriquetral bundles. The dorsal sheaths lie suspended above the

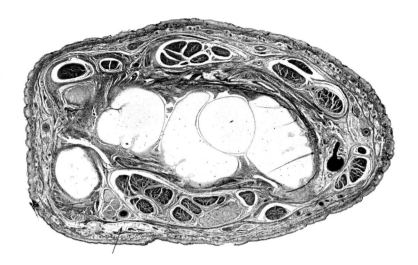

Fig. 1.3 (*series no. 1899*; neg. 15825). Level: 195. Section through the capitate head. Arrow=subcutaneous hypothenar space.

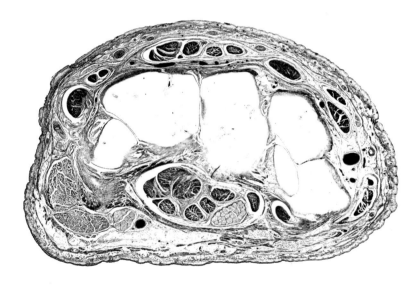

Fig. 1.4 (*series no. 1899*; neg. 13323). Level: 361. Section at distal carpal level.

proximal carpal row. The tuberosity of the scaphoid has moved volar-wards and comes to lie between the flexor carpi radialis and the radial artery, with the result that the radial artery is moved into the dorsal compartment.

4. DISTAL CARPAL LEVEL
(Fig. 1.4.)

The distal carpal bones have developed dorsally to support the now fairly attenuated sheaths of the extensors. The trapezium has extended laterally to support the sheath of the abductor pollicis longus and the extensor pollicis brevis. Actually this sheath is seen to be free at the proximal carpal level and fixed at the distal carpal level. A similar situation prevails for the tendons of the radial extensors of the carpus as they lie above the scaphoid. The dorsal protuberance of the

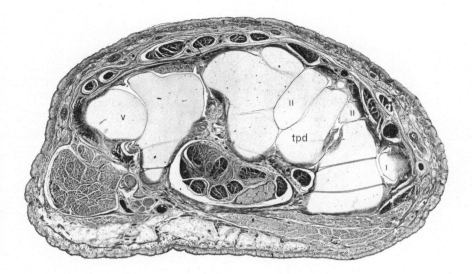

Fig. 1.5 (*series no. 1899*; neg. 16210). Level: 516. Section at the level of carpometacarpal transition. tpd = trapezoid. Roman numerals = the corresponding metacarpals.

trapezoid extends between them and so guides them, as it were, to the bases of the second and third metacarpals. The tendons of the common extensor fan out to form a layer instead of being grouped in a more or less compact mass. The peritendinea reappear while the synovial clefts gradually disappear. The extensor digiti V proprius and the extensor carpi ulnaris are just supported by the lateral extension of the base of the hamate. The flexor retinaculum is now heavily reinforced; it passes beneath the ulnar nerve and vessels. The pisiform has been replaced by the ligamentous column which will divide into the pisohamate and pisometacarpal ligaments. The abductor digiti V is seen in the cross-section. The flexor carpi radialis sheath is firmly attached to the trapezoid. The volar ligaments are nearly all attached to the capitate and to the hamate. Dorsally, the roots of carpo-metacarpal ligaments are visible. Abductor pollicis brevis fascicles have appeared, obviously originating from the tuberosity of the scaphoid. It is necessary to realize that the palmaris longus is more or less part of the fibrous tissue at the base of the thenar eminence, from where extensions can be seen passing into both the flexor retinaculum and the subcorial layers of the skin covering the subcutaneous hypothenar area. The palmaris longus retains a certain individuality.

5. CARPOMETACARPAL TRANSITION ZONE
(Fig. 1.5.)

The radial extensors of the wrist are nearing their insertion. The base of the second metacarpal has appeared on both sides of the trapezoid. The extensor carpi ulnaris has reached the fifth metacarpal. A muscle bundle originates from the hamulus which will separate the deep and superficial branches of the ulnar nerve. Both the radial and ulnar bursae in the carpal tunnel are fully developed. The palmaris brevis has appeared in the section, while the palmar aponeurosis now extends over the thenar eminence.

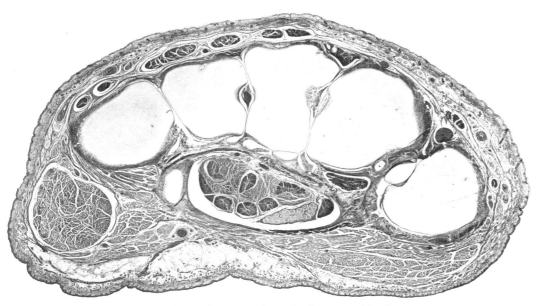

Fig. 1.6 (*series no. 1899*; neg. 13313). Level: 606. Section at basimetacarpal level.

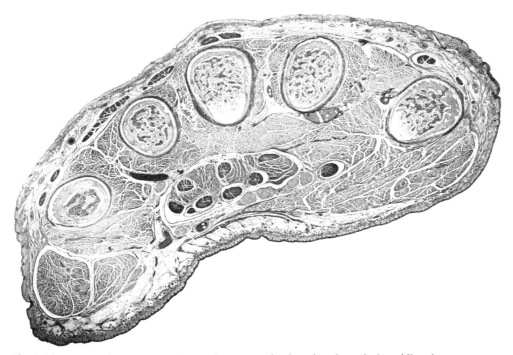

Fig. 1.7 (*series no. 1899*; neg. 13316). Level: 830. Proximal section through the midhand.

6. BASIMETACARPAL LEVEL
(Fig. 1.6.)

The deep ulnar nerve separates the deep and superficial bellies of the opponens digiti V. A fibrous offshoot of the pisometacarpal bundle skirts the hamulus distally en route towards the base of the fourth

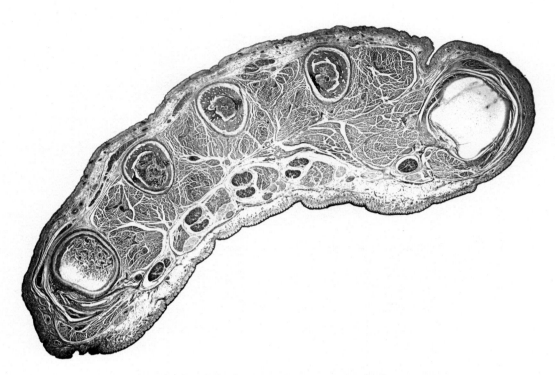

Fig. 1.8 (*series no. 1899*; neg. 13320). Level: 1173. Section halfway through the midhand.

metacarpal. The extensor tendons, except those of the thumb, are all on the *ulnar slope* of the dorsal surface of the metacarpal complex. The flexor carpi radialis is close to its insertion into the second and third metacarpals.

7. PROXIMAL METACARPAL LEVEL
(Fig. 1.7.)
The section is distal to the carpal tunnel. The common digital branch of the ulnar nerve and the ulnar artery can be seen in close apposition to the ulnar bursa. The deep ulnar nerve has just met the perforating artery of the fourth space. A grouping of the superficial and deep tendons of the flexors is imminent.

8. MIDMETACARPAL LEVEL
(Fig. 1.8.)
The gradual retraction of the hypothenar area has brought the flexor tendons closer to the little finger. The widening of the intermetacarpal spaces and the rearrangement of the flexor area have led to the very characteristic widening of this whole area. The deep and superficial tendons of each finger have come closer together; the lumbrical muscles and the common digital nerves occupy the intertendinous areas. The palmar aponeurosis appears largely as a two-layered structure. On the ulnar side the palmar aponeurosis, attached to the

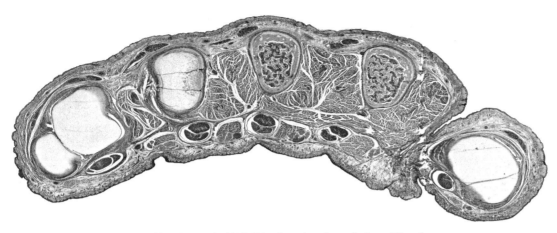

Fig. 1.9 (*series no. 1899*; neg. 22360). Level: 1350. Distal section through the midhand.

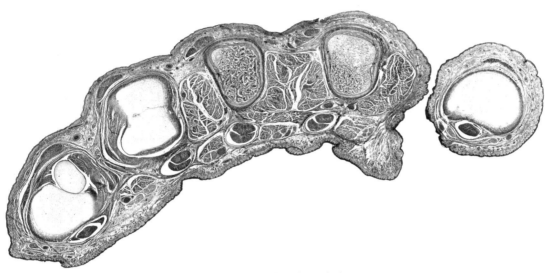

Fig. 1.10 (*series no. 1899*; neg. 22361). Level: 1426. Section through the metacarpophalangeal areas of the fourth and fifth fingers.

hypothenar fascia, closes off the flexor compartment, but on the radial side the compartment is more or less open and faces the subcutaneous thenar space.

9. DISTAL METACARPAL LEVEL
(Fig. 1.9.)
On the ulnar side the interosseous areas are converging towards their respective tendons. Septa derived from the palmar aponeurosis can be seen quite clearly. The distal palmar crease sweeps over the fourth webspace. The metacarpophalangeal segment of the flexor tendon sheath has emerged in the fifth finger.

10. METACARPOPHALANGEAL TRANSITION ZONE
(Fig. 1.10.)
The thumb has become separate from the midhand. Tendons are most

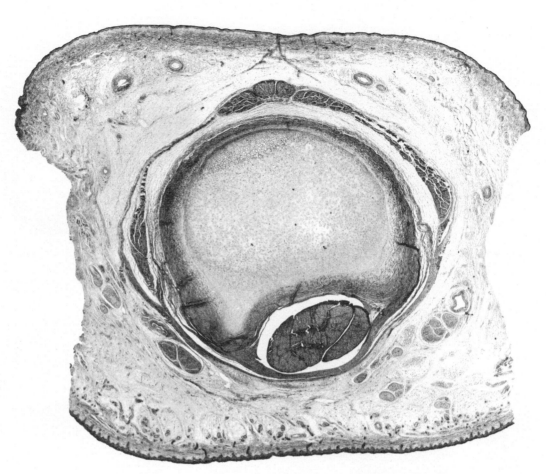

Fig. 1.11 (*series no. 1279*; neg. 21141). Level: 593. Section through the first phalanx just within the palm of the hand. Middle finger. The radial side is at the left.

conspicuous in palmar IV and dorsal IV. The insertion of palmar aponeurosis strands into subcorial layers and the distal termination of its transverse layer have led to the opening of the fourth webspace.

11. PROXIMAL PHALANGEAL LEVEL
(Fig. 1.11.)

The osteofibrous sheath of the first phalanx appears in this section. The fascia around it is continuous proximally with the tendon sheath of the metacarpophalangeal level. Notice the continuity of this fascia with the transverse lamina and also the division into fascicles of the extensor tendon.

12. PROXIMAL INTERPHALANGEAL LEVEL
(Fig. 1.12.)

The fascicles of the extensor assembly can be seen in their typical relation to the phalangeal trochlea. The volar extensions of the extensor assembly are quite conspicuous. The tendon sheath and the palmar pad are suspended from the trochlea of the first phalanx.

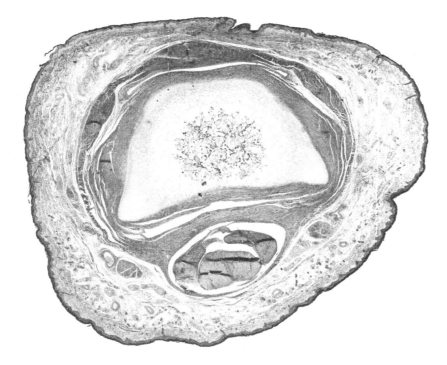

Fig. 1.12 (*series no. 1279*; neg. 21133). Level: 1208. Section through the proximal interphalangeal area.

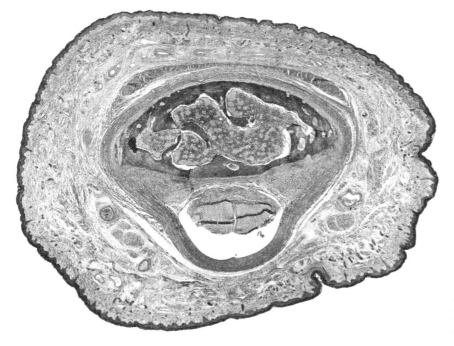

Fig. 1.13 (*series no. 1279*; neg. 21128). Level: 1591. Section through the middle phalanx.

13. MIDDLE PHALANX LEVEL
(Fig. 1.13.)

Again a typical osteofibrous tendon sheath presents. The extensor assembly has lost its centre tendon at the base of this phalanx. Around the sheath an areolar space is bordered by the digital fascia which encloses the digital artery and nerve.

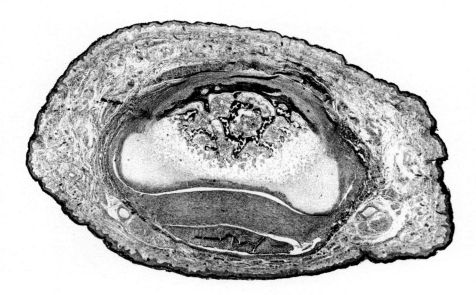

Fig. 1.14 (*series no. 1279*; neg. 21122).
Level: 1809. Section through the distal
interphalangeal area.

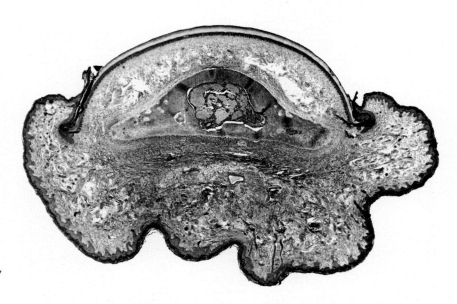

Fig. 1.15 (*series no. 1279*; neg. 21117).
Level: 2253. Section through the tuberosity
of the third phalanx.

14. DISTAL INTERPHALANGEAL LEVEL
(Fig. 1.14.)

The volar plate and the tendon sheath are suspended from the
trochlea of the middle phalanx.

15. THIRD PHALANX LEVEL (TUBEROSITY)
(Fig. 1.15.)

The vault of the nail is supported by fibrous extensions from the
distal tuberosity and the appearance of subdivisions in the volar
pulp is most conspicuous.

The synovial sheath on the ulnar side of the carpal tunnel, the ulnar bursa, soon extends below the deep tendons as far as the tendon for the middle finger. The cleft more or less isolates the deep tendon of the fifth finger and penetrates below the superficial tendons of the fourth and fifth fingers, as well as extending superficially to these tendons. Separate synovial spaces develop in the peritendineum of all superficial tendons (Fig. 2.8).

The situation in Figures 2.6 and 2.7 results quite naturally from the foregoing when account is taken of the processes to which we have already referred. Both the triquetrum and the scaphoid have extended volarwards to such a degree that they provide sites of origin for medially directed ligamentous extensions. Such extensions from the triquetrum retain part of their insertion into the lunate, although the major portion passes this bone distally, as do these ligaments from the scaphoid which originate below the sheath of the flexor carpi radialis. It should be observed also that the ligament from the radius contains a fairly large bundle of rather longitudinal course that also passes the anterior horn of the lunate, this bundle joining the system originating from the scaphoid. Thus there exists a triquetral bundle, radioscaphoidal bundles and bundles of purely scaphoidal origin. These ligamentous strands meet each other distal to the anterior horn of the lunate and therefore in front of the head of the capitate. This happens in such a way that the ligament of the ulnar side splits into two layers and the ligaments from the radial side glide into the resultant fork (Fig. 2.8). This results in the formation of a thick solid ligament layer lying in front of the head of the capitate, a layer that will be invaded distally and replaced by the bases of the hamate and the capitate bones. This results in the formation of the following ligaments, the radioscapho-capitate, the triquetrum-hamate and the hamate-capitate and following retraction of the hamate, of triquetrum-capitate bundles.

In the meantime conspicuous changes have taken place around the pisiform bone. We have already mentioned the emergence of the so-called subcutaneous hypothenar area, a phenomenon which goes with a reinforcement of the fascial layer below the ulnar nerve and vessels, the flexor retinaculum, the layer which is inserted into the pisiform close to its joint cleft with the triquetrum. Close to the distal end of the pisiform two conspicuous bundles radiate medially from the flexor carpi ulnaris-pisiform column, extending like two tongues, one over the flexor retinaculum and the other below the floor of the carpal tunnel. The former bundle fans out distally below the ulnar nerve and vessels (Fig. 2.9); the latter, already visible in Figure 2.8, joins the bundle from the triquetrum. The pisiform being passed, a layer of the flexor retinaculum is seen to continue along the inner side of the fibrous column as the floor of the carpal tunnel (Fig. 2.9). The two tongue-like extensions of the fibrous column distal to the pisiform are both easily visible in the section of Figure 2.10. Note that in this section fibrous strands connect the base of the capitate with the triquetrum and the scaphoid.

The deep pisiform bundle passes to the base of the hamate, as can be seen in Figures 2.11, 2.12 and 2.13, and with the pisiform-hamate column spatially anticipates the hamulus ossis hamati. The superficial pisiform fan becomes engaged in the longitudinal system of the palm

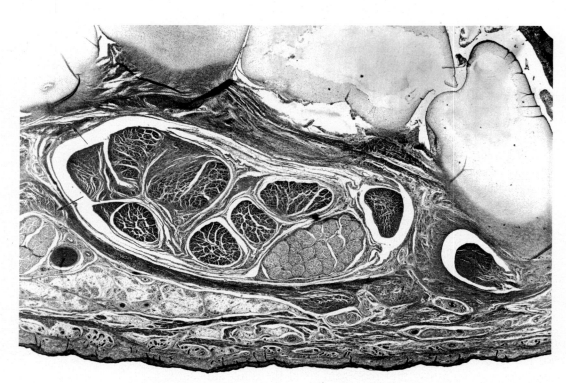

Fig. 2.9 (*series no. 1899*; neg. 13327). Level: 318. The strong ligament layer anterior to the capitate, already locally anchored into the base of the hamate. Note the synovial clefts around the superficial tendons. The tongue-like ligaments radiating from the pisiform column are just visible (arrows).

Fig. 2.10 (*series no. 1899*; neg. 16010). Level: 322. Section through the distal tip of the scaphoid. The ligament originating from the triquetrum (Fig. 2.7, arrow) is inserting now into the hamate (arrow). Both the superficial and deep layers of the extensor communis compartment extend over the dorsal extensors of the wrist and over the extensor pollicis longus. Note the tongue-like ligaments on the inner side of the pisiform and the strong triquetrum capitate bundle. On the inner side of the sheath of the flexor carpi radialis is a strong ligament derived from the flexor retinaculum and the scaphoid tuberosity. This ligament and also the tendon of the abductor, which has deviated from the main bundle, are proximal roots of the abductor pollicis.

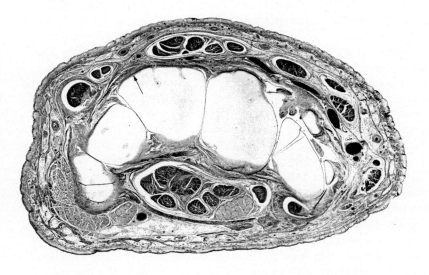

of the hand, the palmar aponeurosis. This is the 'ulnar root' of the palmar aponeurosis which we will discuss in Chapter 4.

We are now quite close to the appearance of the trapezium and the trapezoid and also to the vast extension of the bases of the hamate and the capitate. It seems appropriate now to make some

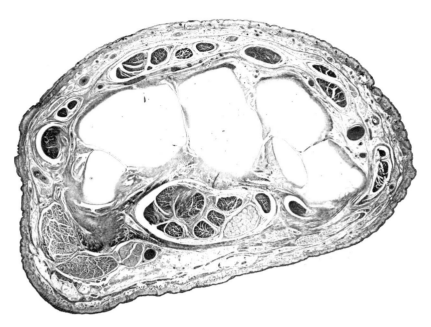

Fig. 2.11 (*series no 1899*; neg. 13323). Level: 361. Section through the distal carpal bases. Both the trapezium and the trapezoid have extended dorsally and so support the sheaths of the abductor pollicis, the extensor pollicis brevis and the laminar system enclosing the radial wrist extensors.

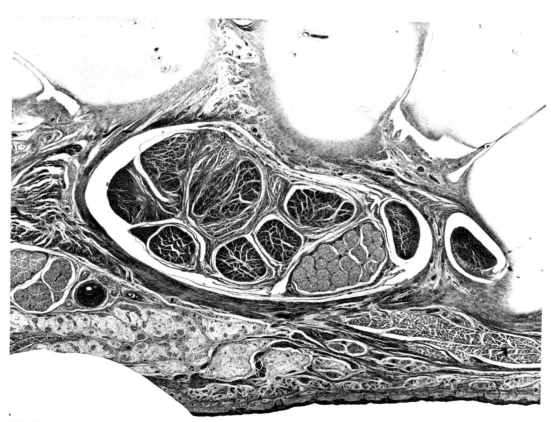

Fig. 2.12 (*series no. 1899*; neg. 13328). Level: 405. The carpal canal at a distal carpal level. Note the insertion of the ulnar wall of the carpal canal into the hamate. The fibrous extension from the sheath of the flexor carpi radialis passing towards the base of the capitate is most conspicuous.

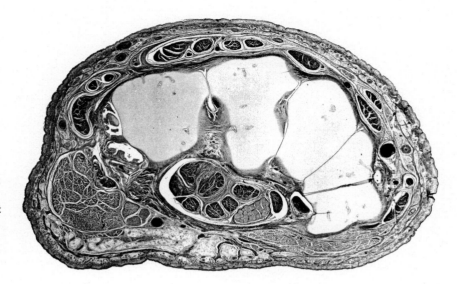

Fig. 2.13 (*series no. 1899*; neg. 16016).
Level: 434. Section through the distal
carpal bases. The fifth metacarpal has just
entered in the section. Note that the
appearance of the opponens pollicis
coincides with a change in cross-section
of the trapezium and with a change in
position of the flexor carpi radialis.

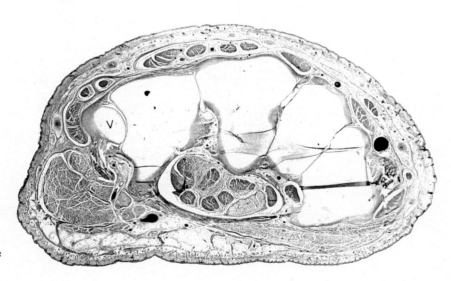

Fig. 2.14 (*series no. 1899*; neg. 16208).
Level: 474. The insertion of the
pisometacarpal bundle into the fifth
metacarpal. The extension of the sheath
of the flexor carpi radialis towards the
capitate base is clearly visible. The radial
fascial extension from the sheaths of the
extensors of the little finger carries the
sheath of the extensor communis and
extends towards the radial extensors of the
wrist. V = the fifth metacarpal.

observations on the position of the sheaths of the extensor carpi
ulnaris and the extensor of the little finger. Comparing Figures 2.5,
2.6 and 2.7 we see a gradual extension of the triquetrum at the
expense of a fibrous area between this bone and the related sheaths.
It can also be established that the superficial fascia is no longer
separated from the sheath proper by an areolar space, for it is now
firmly adherent to this layer. We can also see that the dorsal ligament
strand passing from the triquetrum towards the scaphoid has ended,
and that at the same time another strand has arisen from the triquetrum
which becomes inserted into the hamate bone (Fig. 2.10). The
subsequent retraction of the triquetrum now makes space for the
extending hamate and eventually for the proximal process of metacarpal V and places the associated sheaths in a suspended position
for some distance. It seems that the ligament between the triquetrum

and hamate provides a route for a fibrous extension from the sheaths of the two tendons of the little finger, below the compartment of the extensor communis tendons (Fig. 2.14).

At this point we should note that the latter sheath and the compartment for the extensors carpi radiales and extensor pollicis longus lie in a suspended position over the proximal row. Towards the distal row a slight spreading of the tendon of the extensor communis becomes apparent, with some attenuation of the fibrous loop holding the tendons. The radial extension of the fused layers composing the loop of the communis tendons, passing over the extensors carpi radiales, is similar to the situation found over the proximal row (Figs. 2.4 and 2.5).

The gradual extension of the bases of the distal carpal bones provides bony support for the dorsal tendon layer and leads to the obliteration of the mediocarpal cleft.

We have seen that the radial extensors of the wrist have been displaced to a deeper level and we have seen the deep location of the radial extension of the extensor sheath of the little finger. We have also to take into account the disappearance of the synovial clefts around the radial extensors of the wrist, which means that they come into structural relationship with the fascial layers in which they are embedded. The dorsal extension of the trapezoid extends between the two extensors so that the latter become supported by this bone via the fascial layer between them. The fascial layer between the extensors of the little finger and the radial extensors of the wrist carries the extensor communis tendons, including the indicis proprius, towards the bases of the distal row. The cleft around the ulnar extensor of the wrist is disappearing. The proximal process of the fifth metacarpal emerges just below this tendon and the situation in Figure 2.14 is thus largely explained. In this Figure note: (1) the positions of the radial extensors of the wrist with reference to the trapezoid, (2) the position of the ulnar extensor of the wrist attached to the proximal process of the fifth metacarpal, (3) the position of the lamina extending radially from the sheath of the extensor digiti V below the extensor communis towards the radial extensors of the wrist, (4) the position of the extensor pollicis longus in the superficial fascial layer, (5) an identical situation for the short extensor of the thumb, (6) the bony support for the abductor pollicis longus, and (7) note that the latter muscle comes close to its insertion by the disappearance of the synovial cleft around this tendon.

It is quite obvious that other changes are taking place at the levels under consideration. The pisiform area is transformed into a fibrous mass that concentrates in two main extensions, (1) a pisiform-hamulus bundle, with the two tongues, and (2) a thick pisometacarpal ligament. The latter will be seen to find its main insertion in the anterior and ulnar aspects of the fifth metacarpal, the most external bundles merging with the inserting ulnar extensor of the wrist. One fascicle, in close apposition to the hamulus, skirts this process distally and will be seen to become inserted into the fourth metacarpal. The space between the two main extensions of the ligamentous pisiform column leads to the capsule of the triquetrum-hamate joint.

The fibrous corona around the pisiform area serves as the area of origin of the abductor digiti V, which soon forms a large area anterior

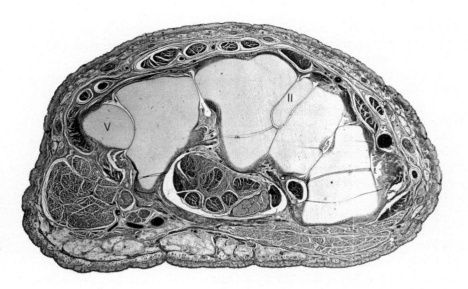

Fig. 2.15 (*series no. 1899*; neg. 16209). Level: 496. Part of the base of the second metacarpal has appeared in the section and shows a slip from the bifurcated ligament from the trapezoid inserted into it. A muscular bundle originates from the tip of the hamulus. II = the second metacarpal; V = the fifth metacarpal.

to the pisiform. The pisometacarpal ligament lies in the floor of this area.

The ulnar nerve divides into two branches over the hamulus ossis hamati. The deep branch follows the inner pisometacarpal strand that skirts the distal aspect of the hamulus. Pisometacarpal bundles approach the anterior aspect of the fifth metacarpal (Figs. 2.15 and 2.16) and subsequently a fibrous strand emerges between the side of the tip of the hamulus and the fifth metacarpal (Fig. 2.16). This extension runs below the deep branch of the ulnar nerve and the abductor and it covers the pisometacarpal bundles mentioned above. Another fibrous extension originates from the very tip of the hamulus which separates the two main divisions of the ulnar nerve.

Both fibrous arches from the hamulus are related to muscle compartments. The deep arch is the proximal border of the deep compartment of the opponens; the superficial arch is the proximal reinforced border of a muscular compartment that holds the superficial opponens portion and a muscular bundle that will join the abductor, as will be seen in another chapter. The position of the deep branch of the ulnar nerve between two muscular compartments, viz. the deep opponens and the superficial opponens can be clearly seen in Figure 2.18.

The proximal extension of the thenar musculature, apparently the abductor pollicis, is rooted in an extremely dense fibrous system around the sheath of the flexor carpi radialis, anchored with the sheath into the scaphoid tuberosity and structurally intimately interconnected with the flexor retinaculum which forms an integral part of the local subcorial system. The scaphoid moves so far volarwards that only a few fascial laminae intervene between this protuberance and the subcorial layer. This same area sees the origin of a longitudinal bundle that is seen more distally as a twin bundle, or a satellite bundle, of the palmaris longus. Its origin is found in the scaphoid tuberosity mainly deep to the sheath of the flexor carpi radialis, while fibres from the tip of the tuberosity pass over the tendon towards this longitudinal bundle (Figs. 2.7, 2.8 and 2.9) which

Fig. 2.16 (*series no. 1899*; neg. 16211).
Level: 538. The base of the second
metacarpal has extended considerably.
The other slip of the bifurcated ligament
from the trapezoid is seen to be inserted
into it. The bases of metacarpals I, III and
IV have now appeared next to II and V.
Notice the strand below the abductor
digiti V. It represents the proximal
border of the deep opponens compartment
(cf. Fig. 2.18). Roman numerals indicate
the corresponding metacarpals. ham =
hamate; cap = capitate; tpd = trapezoid;
tpm = trapezium; p.o.l. = posterior
oblique ligament; x = proximal origin
interossei; a.o.l. = anterior oblique
ligament.

is a proximal tendon of the abductor pollicis brevis. Other fascicles of
the muscle arise from the fibrous system over the sheath and it can be
seen that one tiny tendon of the abductor longus serves as a tendon
of origin for the abductor brevis.

Quite soon we see two parts of the most proximal origin of the
opponens pollicis below the abductor, (1) from the lateral aspect of
the trapezium (Fig. 2.13) and (2) from the adjoining deep layer of the
flexor retinaculum (Fig. 2.14).

Screening of the sections beyond the levels of the scaphoid
tuberosity again particularly shows the fibrous system between the
trapezium and the capitate base, a system that includes the sheath of
the flexor carpi radialis and, as can be seen in Figure 2.11, this system
is an entity in itself extending from the trapezium towards the
capitate base. This system is situated distal to the medio-distally
directed ligaments between scaphoid and capitate (Fig. 2.9). It appears
now that this sheath moves gradually deeper so that the tuberosity
of the trapezium overhangs the sheath to some degree. The result is
that eventually the sheath becomes lodged in the niche between
trapezium and trapezoid. The main anchor of the sheath dependent
fibrous system into the capitate is now replaced by another (Fig. 2.13),
which finds a strong insertion into the trapezoid (Fig. 2.16), an
attachment which serves as a fulcrum for the tendon of the flexor
carpi radialis. This system is reinforced by fibres derived from the
flexor retinaculum that constitute the radial wall of the carpal canal
and also by fibres from the trapezium running dorsal to the tendon
of the flexor carpi radialis (Fig. 2.17). In Figure 2.18 this ligament
represents a fairly separate structure. As soon as the trapezium-
metacarpal I joint cleft appears in the section and also the cleft
between trapezoid and the second metacarpal, the system in which
the tendon of the carpi radialis is caught becomes somewhat
suspended. It is obvious that this is only transitory as the clefts are
soon passed and will lead to a gradual apposition of both the deep
ligament and the tendon to the second metacarpal (Fig. 2.20). The

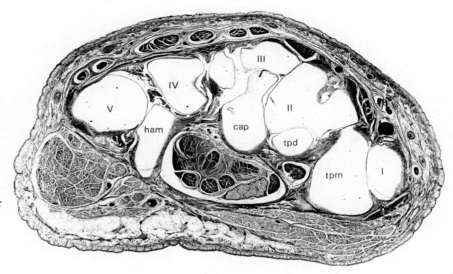

Fig. 2.17 (*series no. 1899*; neg. 16212).
Level: 544. Section through the hamulus.
Note the fibres between hamulus and
capitate and the deep ligaments between
trapezium, trapezoid and capitate. In the
hypothenar area the fascial strand from
hamulus to the fifth metacarpal and a
fascial strand from this bone that merges
with the abductor fascia are clearly
visible. The latter strand contains muscular
bundles from the tip of the hamulus.
Roman numerals indicate the respective
metacarpals. ham = hamate; cap =
capitate; tpd = trapezoid; tpm =
trapezium.

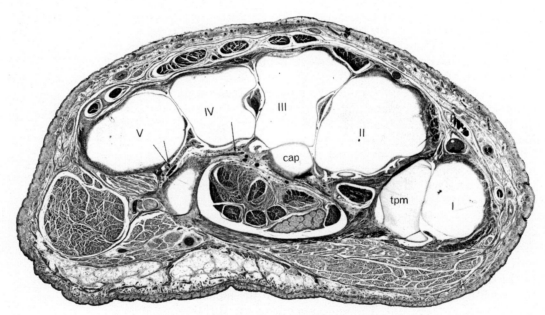

Fig. 2.18 (*series no. 1899*; neg. 13312). Level: 580. Section through the metacarpal bases.
The trapezium is still in the cross-section. Note the fibrous system surrounding the
flexor carpi radialis tendon. The arrow points to the ligament from the base of the
hamulus. The double stemmed arrow indicates the medial slip of the pisometacarpal
complex. Note the deep ulnar nerve between the two muscular areas. The wing-like
radial extension of the sheath of the extensors of the little finger passes below the
extensor communis. The thenar musculature, opponens and abductor extend well over
the flexor retinaculum. Roman numerals indicate the corresponding metacarpals. cap =
capitate; tpm = trapezium.

insertion of the flexor carpi radialis into the second metacarpal with
a slip into the third, is easily seen in Figure 2.21.

We should mention here that the ulnar wall of the carpal tunnel
continues distally as an intramuscular septum, which becomes
firmly anchored to the fifth metacarpal. This septum which is the

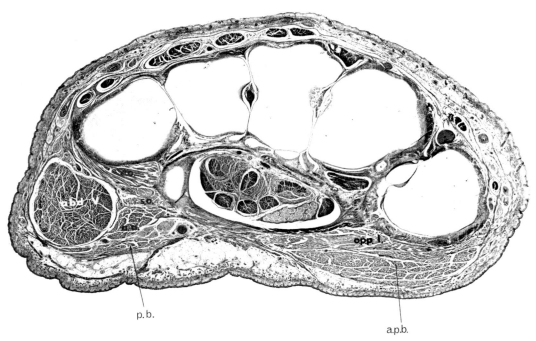

Fig. 2.19 (*series no. 1899*; neg. 13313). Level: 606. Section through the metacarpal base. Note the strand running medially from the hamulus with the pisometacarpal bundle below it. The deep ulnar nerve runs between the two opponens layers. The abductor pollicis longus is now firmly anchored to the metacarpal base. The abductor pollicis brevis has just slightly retracted its medial border. The double layer encasing the extensors of the little finger also encloses the tendons of the extensor communis. opp. I = opponens pollicis; abd. = abductor digiti V; d.o. = deep opponens layer; s.o. = superficial opponens layer; a.a. = additional abductor bundle; p.b. = palmaris brevis; a.p.b. = abductor pollicis brevis.

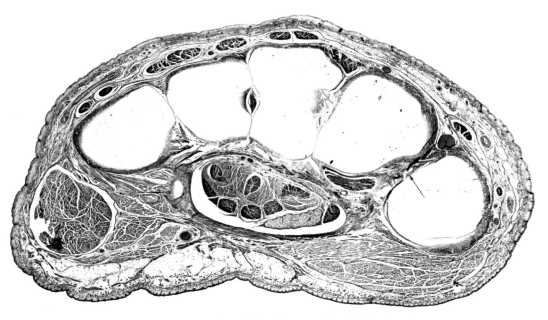

Fig. 2.20 (*series no. 1899*; neg. 13314). Level: 632. The flexor carpi radialis is close to its insertion. The first adductor bundles appear in the floor of the carpal canal. The area of origin of palmar I becomes apparent in the fibrous system around the flexor carpi radialis. Arrow = insertion of the posterior oblique ligament.

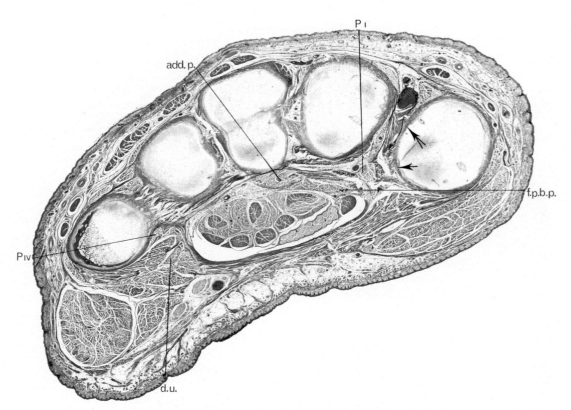

Fig. 2.21 (*series no. 1899*; neg. 13315). Level: 694. Section through the distal level of the carpal canal. Fibrous radiations from the palmaris brevis which pass into the hypothenar skin are quite conspicuous. The superficial tendons are each surrounded by a synovial sheath. The most distal fibres of the posterior oblique ligament of the thumb are indicated by a double stemmed arrow. P I = m.interosseus palmaris I; P IV = m.interosseus palmaris IV; f.p.b.p. = flexor pollicis brevis profundus; add.p = adductor pollicis; d.u. = deep branch of the ulnar nerve; arrow = anterior oblique ligament.

distal continuity of the hamulus and is soon replaced by another, serves as the site of origin of palmar IV. In the case of a movable metacarpal, such as the first metacarpal, a firm flexor tunnel anchorage by an intramuscular septum is hardly feasible. As shown in Figure 2.21 the core of the fibrous system (Fig. 2.20), anterior to the flexor carpi radialis, is gradually replaced by a muscle that might be distinguished as the first palmar interosseus. Both the adductor and the deep flexor pollicis brevis are related to the floor of the carpal tunnel.

Further observations of the carpometacarpal transition will be made later, but here we should mention some phenomena which might otherwise be neglected.

The emergence of the hamulus ossis hamati is anticipated by the pisiform-hamate column and the tongue-like ligament below the floor of the carpal tunnel while the insertion of this ligament into the hamate spatially forecasts the appearance of the hamulus. A ligament extends medially from the distal aspect of the base of this process and again we have a fibrous layer representing the floor of the tunnel (Figs. 2.19 and 2.20). This layer meets its counterpart anterior to the third metacarpal, to which they are both anchored. Below this layer, on the radial side, runs the flexor carpi radialis tendon which is inserted eventually into the second and third metacarpals. Below the ulnar area runs a small ligament, the medial bundle of the pisometa-carpal complex (Fig. 2.20). This bundle will become inserted into the base of the fourth metacarpal.

Towards the bases of the distal carpal bones the synovial clefts in the carpal tunnel still extend over a considerable distance. It seems even that the two bursae have approached each other on the volar aspect just as the ulnar bursa now also nearly touches the median nerve. Clefts can still be seen around the superficial tendons. Towards the end of the carpal canal the ulnar bursa slightly retracts from below the deep tendons IV and V. The cleft between the profundus tendons IV and V becomes closed off towards the ulnar bursa, so that the cleft between these tendons will come to end blindly.

The sheath of the sublimis tendon V is an extremely thin structure (Fig. 2.12) which opens towards the ulnar bursa at about the level in Figure 2.13. The reclosure of the sheath is observed at levels just distal to Figure 2.14. In Figure 2.15 this cleft is seen closed towards the ulnar bursa.

2. CARPOMETACARPAL TRANSITION

Carpometacarpal transition is embodied in fairly gradually progres-sing phenomena and we have already seen various phenomena which have anticipated this transition. Among these we may mention the changes going on in the dorsal tendon sheaths which can be described as the transition of sheaths proper into laminar suspension layers of the extensor tendons. Another marked phenomenon concerns the shaping of the bases of the distal carpal bones to conform to the shape of bases of the metacarpals. Wedging of the distal carpal bases is clearly visible in Figure 2.13.

We have already pointed out the appearance of the proximal process of the fifth metacarpal in the dorsal concavity on the lateral aspect of the hamate. The volar facet was occupied by a distal extension of the triquetrum. The proximal extension of the first metacarpal appears at the same levels in the conspicuous dent on the dorsal side of the trapezium. Figure 2.13 shows these phenomena and the same figure provides clear evidence of the ligamentous bridging of the intercarpal joint clefts on their dorsal sides. It is perhaps useful to be reminded here of those dorsal ligaments which were observed between the triquetrum and the hamate at more proximal levels and also of the dorsal ligaments between the trapezium and trapezoideum and between the latter and the capitate which can be seen in Figure 2.13.

The origins of some of the ligaments in Figure 2.13 are to be seen in Figure 2.11. These latter dorsal ligaments are represented at more distal levels by the carpometacarpal ligaments. The origins of these ligaments and their insertions represent the conspicuous phenomena in Figure 2.15 and subsequent sections. In these sections the second metacarpal is seen firmly anchored to the base of the trapezoid by means of bifurcating ligaments. It seems to be very appropriate to point out an extremely conspicuous ligament that is seen to originate in Figure 2.16 from the ulnar aspect of the capitate and that is also observed in Figure 2.18 to run distally in an interosseal niche, between the third and fourth metacarpals. This ligament will eventually become inserted into the ulnar aspect of the base of the third metacarpal. This ligament obviously represents a longitudinal interosseal carpometacarpal junction and is unique of its kind.

Deep palmar anchorages exist between the bases of the hamulus and capitate (Fig. 2.16) which represent a deep division of the mediodistally running ulnar ligament system. Distal to the hamulus they are replaced by a bundle passing from the distal aspect of the hamulus to the third metacarpal (Fig. 2.18) and subsequently by the medial bundle of the pisometacarpal ligament, the bundle which skirts the hamulus distally (Fig. 2.20) and is inserted into the base of the fourth metacarpal. Deep palmar anchorages also exist between the capitate and the trapezoid (Fig. 2.14) and between the trapezoid and the trapezium (Fig. 2.16). These ligaments form part of or are identical to the ligamentous system around the tendon of the flexor carpi radialis of which we have spoken earlier in this chapter.

We wish to draw special attention to a strong ligamentous root on the ulnodorsal aspect of the trapezium (Fig. 2.15). Careful analysis of this area proves that what we are seeing here is the root of the posterior oblique ligament of the first carpometacarpal joint. This ligament can be followed in subsequent sections as far as its insertion into the ulnar aspect of the base of the first phalanx (Fig. 2.21). This same figure shows intermetacarpal ligaments present between the various metacarpals and particularly between the first and second. Figure 2.19 shows a dense fibrous collar around the base of the first metacarpal. The abductor pollicis longus tendon can easily be traced as far as its insertion. Further the anterior oblique ligament of the first carpometacarpal joint is to be sought in this collar. Its origin from the volar tubercle of the trapezium has been indicated in Figure 2.16 and its insertion into the first metacarpal can be seen in Figure 2.21.

A fibrous strand below the radial artery, visible in Figure 2.16, extends into the area of origin of the radial belly of the first dorsal interosseus, while another strand also below this artery, shown in Figure 2.16, has split off from the tendon of the extensor carpi radialis longus and extends towards the volar side, serving the first palmar interosseus as tendon of origin.

We have now virtually arrived at the proximal base of the midhand. It may be appropriate to point out some features of the base of the metacarpal region, which can be seen in Figures 2.18, 2.19 and 2.20. It is obvious that the situation here is much simpler than that found at carpal levels. The carpal muscles have found their insertion and we have to consider only the extensors and flexors of the digits. The arrangement of the extensors in the midhand can be understood by taking into account the disappearance of the synovial clefts, a phenomenon accompanied by a marked attenuation of the fibrous loops and rings at carpal level and the emergence of peritendineal layers. As Figure 2.18 shows, the extensors of the little finger, each still surrounded by a synovial cleft, pass through a fibrofascial layer that extends both in radial and ulnar directions. In the ulnar direction the layer is firmly anchored to the base of the fifth metacarpal, while in the radial direction the layer extends below that of the extensor communis, incorporating a strong ligament which originates from the base of the capitate and which is seen to become inserted into the base of the fourth metacarpal. It appears that this layer extends radially beyond the ligament over the third metacarpal, so providing a cover for the tendons of both the long and short radial extensors of the wrist. These tendons are close to their insertion and it seems worthwhile to observe that these tendons and the ligament passing towards the fourth metacarpal are in much the same anatomical position.

A similar picture prevails for the common extensors of the digits. The tendons are held in a fascial layer that we can now describe as an intertendineal fascia. This layer is naturally derived from the peritendineum and is covered by a supratendineal fascia derived from the superficial layer of the fibrous loop surrounding the extensor communis. It blends ulnarwards with the layer over the tendons of the little finger. On following this layer radially it is seen to divide twice to enclose successively the long and short extensors of the thumb.

An areolar space exists under the supratendineal layer and another space separates this layer from the subcutaneous layers. The former space becomes obliterated towards the thenar and hypothenar eminences. In the chapter on the midhand we will see a blending of the subcutaneous fascia with the superficial or supratendineal layer, as a result of which the areolar space between the inter- and supratendineal layers becomes the 'gliding' space between the skin and subjacent tendineal structures. A similar situation prevails in the fingers.

Another phenomenon which to a certain extent determines the basimetacarpal situation is seen in the appearance of the thenar and hypothenar eminences and the subcutaneous hypothenar area. These developments will be discussed in the appropriate chapters.

DISCUSSION

It need hardly be emphasized that it would be most rewarding to find a way of fitting the collected data into a coherent system, so that the carpal region could be assessed easily in an analytical manner and could be explored on the basis of such a coherent analytical plan.

The first point to be decided about this area is that it is not an area of gradual transitions but an area which links together basically different regions, i.e. the forearm and the hand. It is obvious that the proximal carpal row establishes this link while the distal row can be looked upon as a proximal base of the midhand. Although the appearance of the distal row reflects the fan-like arrangement of the hand, this view is not applicable to the structure of the proximal row. A basic feature of the proximal row, including the head of the capitate, is the shape of the individual bones and their mutual positions as seen in cross-section. The spherical surfaces of scaphoid, lunate, capitate and triquetrum have been mentioned repeatedly and we have also pointed out that the ligamentous relationships of the proximal carpal bones can be understood by taking into account their positions with respect to both dorsal and volar ligament layers, which present as the distal extensions of the dorsal and palmar borders of the radius.

The fact that both scaphoid and lunate do not extend dorsally to touch the dorsal tendon-carrying ligament layer makes it possible for arterial branches to pass into the subtendineal space over the proximal row. The firm anchorage of the anterior horn of the lunate to the anterior ligaments is a marked phenomenon and so is the anterior extension of the scaphoid tuberosity. The anterior location of the scaphoid tuberosity between the tendon of the flexor carpi radialis and the radial artery leads the latter into the 'tabatière anatomique', a space that becomes apparent distal to the styloid process of the radius. Moreover, the anterior extension of this bone creates an origin for mediodistally running ligaments. The position of the triquetrum is certainly not a mirror image of that of the scaphoid. While the latter bone virtually retracts from the dorsal tendon layer (Figs. 2.4 and 2.5) as already pointed out, the triquetrum extends into the dorsal ligament layer and so becomes the site of attachment for dorsal radiocarpal ligaments and the site of origin of a ligamentous strand extending over the carpus distally towards the scaphoid (Fig. 2.5). In addition, the triquetrum itself extends distal to the volar ulnocarpal ligament and in a palmar direction into the palmar fibrous layer in the same manner as the lunate, with the result that a strong band is seen between the two bones (Fig. 2.7). The contribution from the triquetrum to the band in front of the capitate head can be understood from this palmar extension of the bone. Dorsally and laterally the triquetrum invades the ligamentous layer so that the triquetrum is a marked stronghold for much of the ligamentous system of the carpus.

A Figure such as 2.5 gives some idea of a mechanical and functional unit within the carpus, the complex composed of the capitate head enclosed by the lunate and scaphoid, with the triquetrum as a keystone of an auxiliary ligamentous system.

We have already spoken of the arrangement at basimetacarpal levels, an arrangement which was anticipated at distal carpal levels. We would like to point out the spreading and flattening of the dorsal tendons, the dorsal extension of the distal carpal bones and the wedging of their bases (Figs. 2.13 and 2.14). These features can be related to the marked curvature of the distal carpal region as seen in these figures. The distal carpal bones collectively establish an arched structure. In comparison the situation is totally different on the palmar aspect. Instead of the laminated arrangement of fascias and tendons of the dorsal side we see a dense interweaving of skin with subjacent layers, forming a subcorial fibrous system, beneath which lie the thenar and hypothenar fascias and with which firm attachments exist (Fig. 2.10).

This fibrous structural system of the palmar side forms a more or less flat base for the dorsal vault of the carpus. The picture of the fibrous structure becomes more marked when we look at the carpal eminences (the pisiform and hamulus and the scaphoid and trapezium) and the strong fibrous flexor retinacular system between these eminences, particularly between the distal eminences. The strong dorsal arching of the distal carpal bones goes hand-in-hand with the development of a strong flexor retinaculum. In this respect it is quite intriguing to observe the position of the carpal eminences, again the distal ones in particular, for on comparison with the styloid processes of radius and ulna we see that the distal eminences are placed more internally with the specific result that the dorsal arching is combined with considerable reinforcement of the palmar base.

A basic feature of the palmar aspect of the carpal region seems to be the tendency of ligaments to converge towards the midline of the hand. The radiocarpal and ulnocarpal ligaments display this behaviour quite strikingly, but hardly less than the ligaments originating from (1) the tuberosities of the scaphoid and the trapezium, (2) the triquetrum and (3) the base of the hamulus.

It is quite remarkable that the carpal flexors join the medially directed trend. The flexor carpi radialis curves medially through a tunnel derived from the trapezium and one which is firmly inserted into the trapezoid. On the ulnar side the flexor carpi ulnaris continues distally beyond the pisiform as the pisohamate and the pisometa-carpal ligaments. One of the strands of this ligament skirts the hamu-lus on its anterior aspect and joins the medially directed layer of ligaments. One can imagine such a system being derived from a transverse system by the distal displacement of a medial anchorage. Such a process would involve neither the dorsal ligament system nor the palmar system of the flexor retinaculum, because neither of these two finds an anchorage in the midline of the hand, as does the deep volar system. The longitudinal systems of both the flexors and extensors of the digits, as well as the palmaris longus, cross the basic transverse system of the carpus.

It becomes urgent now to comment upon the carpal eminences placed on the inner side of the distal continuations of the styloid processes of radius and ulna. In the radial column lined up one behind the other, we see the scaphoid tuberosity, the trapezium and the first metacarpal; the tendon of the flexor carpi radialis runs on the inner side of this column, but on the ulnar side a continuous osseous column does not exist. On the ulnar side an osteofibrous column may be determined by the continuation of the tendon of flexor carpi ulnaris. This column would comprise the pisiform bone, the piso-hamate and pisometacarpal ligaments and finally the hamulus. On the other hand it can be seen that the pisiform continues distally into a muscular column of the abductor digiti V. When we compare the course of the carpal flexors it becomes apparent that both tendons converge to the midline of the hand, the radial flexor in its entirety, the ulnar flexor by one of the slips of the pisometacarpal ligament only.

As we have seen the hamulus serves as a fulcrum for this tendon fascicle and so ensures the bend in its course. Considering the positions of the hamulus and of the fibrous structures which antici-pate this bony eminence proximally, we may say that the tendon fascicle skirts the ulnar wall of the flexor tendon compartment. The radial carpal flexor displays much the same arrangement, for it too skirts a fibrous wall, i.e. the radial wall of the flexor compartment. There are a number of consequences arising from these points.

Firstly, while the flexor carpi radialis is seen to run outside the carpal tunnel this tendon actually skirts the radial wall of the tunnel. Secondly, the osseous support of the carpal tunnel is entirely com-posed of the hamulus ossis hamati. Thirdly, the radial carpal emin-ence has its corollary in a column consisting of the pisiform bone and the abductor digiti V. Lastly the attachment of the carpal tunnel to the scaphoid and especially to the trapezium provides a kind of secondary anchorage. These bones are not truly incorporated in the carpal tunnel as is the hamulus.

SUMMARY

The functional-spatial concept that has been applied throughout this analysis has provided a considerably simplified view of carpal structure.

The most essential point in carpal structure is the linkage of two different regions, the lower arm and the hand (including the distal carpal bones). The linkage system consists of the proximal carpal bones and the scaphoid, lunate and capitate represent the key-linkage mechanism.

The lunate is anchored firmly in a ligament system which represents the continuity of the anterior border of radius and triangular disc. This ligament layer is continued distally by contributions from the scaphoid, trapezium and triquetrum. This ligament layer runs freely in front of the head of the capitate. The bases of hamate and capitate are firmly anchored to this layer.

The dorsal ligament layer is anchored to the triquetrum. By dorsal and lateral extension this latter bone supports the tendon sheaths of the extensor carpi ulnaris and the extensor of the little finger. The dorsal tendons pass into a suspended position just over the proximal carpal bones; because of the central location of these bones, they are also supported by the bases of the distal carpal bones. The dorsal passage of the radial artery and its branches is dependent upon the position of suspension of these tendons.

The fibrous loops and rings which pass round the synovial sheaths of the extensor tendons are anchored to the radius and their position is related to the course of the tendons.

The relation of the sheath of the extensor carpi ulnaris to the ulna is most typical. The transition of tendon sheaths into tendon layers (a process that takes place over the bases of distal carpal bones) involves the attenuation of the fibrous constituents of the tendon sheath; the disappearance of clefts coincides with the reappearance of intertendineal masses that become intertendineal layers and are suspended below the supratendineal fascial layer which in turn is derived from the fibrous loops and rings. The carpal tunnel is a fibrous structure supported mainly by the hamulus, a bony eminence virtually incorporated in the tunnel wall. The radial wall of this tunnel is anchored to the tuberosity of the trapezium through exchange of fibres between the flexor retinaculum and the sheath of the flexor carpi radialis.

The radial carpal eminence represents a column carrying the first ray of the hand. It is composed of the scaphoid tuberosity, the trapezium and the first metacarpal. Its contralateral corollary is embodied in the pisiform, extending distally in the abductor digiti V. On the ulnar side a part of the distal extension of the carpal flexor (viz. the pisohamate ligament) merges with the ulnar wall of the flexor compartment.

In the coming paragraphs on the midhand some further points will be made concerning the importance of the hamulus in the origin of hypothenar and thenar musculature and the significance of the carpal tunnel wall as the site of origin of thenar musculature.

3. The Midhand

This chapter concerns the metacarpal region from the carpus to the phalanges and includes an analysis of the separate columns in the hand, viz. the thenar, the hypothenar and the interossei. In this chapter due attention is given to the general arrangement of this region, the mutual relationships of various structures, the course of the extensor tendons and the grouping of the flexor tendons. We present a survey of the region in two separate paragraphs 1 and 3 respectively, which cover the proximal and distal palmar areas. Those paragraphs are based on an analysis of the transverse *series no. 1899*. Paragraph 2 relates to the separate columns of the hand which were first examined in *series no. 1452* and later in *series no. 1899* and the analysis is given here in this order.

1. THE PROXIMAL MIDHAND AREA

We chose a section through the zone of transition between carpus and metacarpus to provide a proximal base for our study (Fig. 2.18). The section closely approaches the distal border of the hamulus. A pisometacarpal bundle will soon skirt the anterior (distal) aspect on its way to the base of the fourth metacarpal. The flexor carpi radialis tendon is in a very similar position as it passes to the bases of the second and third metacarpals. The small tips of the bases of the capitate and trapezium are the only carpal remnants in the section.

At this level we see a fibrous area which represents the distal continuity of the tuberosity of the trapezium. Extensions from this column in a medial direction radiate into the flexor retinaculum and radial extensions from this latter layer provide both wall and floor of the carpal canal. This extension, passing on the inner aspect of the flexor carpi radialis tendon, maintains a position comparable to that of the hamulus since it forms a lateral wall of the tunnel.

In a section such as Figure 2.19, in which the base of the capitate bone is on the point of disappearing from the section, we see the most distal strand of the ligament lying between the hamulus and the capitate base, which does not become inserted into this base but passes to the base of the third metacarpal. This ligamentous strand is joined by the pisometacarpal bundle, which, because of its deeper position, will be arrested by the base of the fourth metacarpal. Radially, the base of the third metacarpal is approached by the extensions of the flexor retinaculum which run on the palmar aspect of the flexor carpi radialis and which, in more proximal sections, are seen to be inserted into the base of the capitate bone and into the trapezoid, the latter serving as a fulcrum for the flexor carpi radialis (Fig. 2.17).

The radial and ulnar bursae show virtually their greatest extension in the carpal canal, where these two bursae actually touch an extremely loose areolar space lying over the median nerve. The radial bursa entirely surrounds the flexor pollicis longus. The ulnar bursa has an extension lying between the superficial tendons of the fourth and fifth fingers on the one hand and the deep tendon of the fifth finger and its lumbrical on the other. The superficial tendons are each surrounded by a synovial cleft. The cleft around the superficial tendon of the little finger communicated proximally with the ulnar bursa (Fig. 2.14) and is reduced here to a small cavity. This tendon is attached to the peritendineum of the neighbouring tendon in a peculiar manner, which can be particularly well seen in Figure 3.2.

The thenar eminence is already considerably extended, for the abductor pollicis and the opponens are both visible. The abductor digiti V, the two parts of the opponens and the abductor portion originating from the hamulus (Fig. 2.20) can all be identified in the hypothenar eminence.

The subcutaneous hypothenar compartment is a conspicuous feature at these levels, as is the palmaris brevis with its skin anchorages. The palmar aponeurosis is already spreading out and the flexor retinaculum contributes substantially to this layer.

The extensor tendons are in quite a characteristic position. The tendons of the little finger, each of them still surrounded by a synovial cleft, are held in a layer which, on the ulnar side, merges with the hypothenar compartment wall or with the periosteum of the fifth metacarpal. At carpal levels on the radial side it can be seen that this tendon-holding layer, over its major part, continues as an infra-tendinous layer below the extensor communis and so merges with the layer of the radial extensors of the wrist (cf. Fig. 2.15). At the basimetacarpal level (Figs. 2.19 and 2.20) we find that the extensor digiti V covering layer also extends superficially to the extensor tendons of the fingers. It appears that this situation becomes the prevailing one at metacarpal levels, which means that the digiti V extensor and the common finger extensors become embedded in one double layer. This situation does not prevent the extensors of the little finger from maintaining their own compartments within this layer (Fig. 2.19). In this same figure we can see that the extensors of the thumb are embedded in the supratendinous layer which extends radially from above the extensor communis.

On comparing Figures 2.19 and 2.21, it would appear that the fibrous area constituting the radial wall and the adjacent floor of the flexor tunnel becomes replaced by the adductor pollicis. A deep core of this fibrous area gives rise to a muscular bundle just anterior to the first metacarpal and this bundle may be identified as palmar interosseus I. In these same sections the extension of both the opponens pollicis and the abductor pollicis brevis is quite conspicuous. A large area of the flexor retinaculum becomes replaced by the opponens pollicis, which was seen to occur at more proximal carpal levels for the abductor brevis.

For the detailed constitution of the hypothenar eminence we would refer the reader to the relative paragraph. Now that the hamulus has been passed it is sufficient to note that both the deep opponens layer and the area comprising the superficial opponens and the additional abductor have appeared in the cross-section.

The section under consideration (Fig. 2.21) has also touched upon the most proximal bundles of some of the interossei, those of dorsal I and dorsal IV and the very conspicuous origin of palmar IV in the outer niche of the ulnar wall of the carpal tunnel. This situation deserves attention as it is related to the imminent passage of the deep branch of the ulnar nerve into the deep palmar space.

Figure 3.1 shows the dissolution of the ulnar wall of the carpal tunnel, which makes the way free for the deep branch of the ulnar nerve to pass towards the deeper regions. Further distally a new ulnar flexor compartment wall is formed; this wall, however, extends into an intramuscular septum between palmar IV and the opponens digiti V (Fig. 3.7). Thus the passage of the nerve goes with the displacement of a muscle from the exterior to the interior of a compartment.

Future sections will show us the proximal origins of interossei, the passage of the deep ulnar nerve through the adductor, the passage of the deep palmar arch through this same muscle and the emergence of the superficial bellies of the flexor pollicis brevis.

It is obvious that identification of interosseous areas, as they appear at these basimetacarpal levels, can only be achieved by using information present at more distal levels. At a level such as that of Figure 3.11 the interosseous areas can be clearly defined from each other. Palmar IV represents a quadrangular field at the radiopalmar aspect of metacarpal V. Dorsal IV occupies the major part of the fourth intermetacarpal space and its volar tip moves between palmar IV and palmar III towards the deep palmar fascia. Palmar III, in its turn, occupies the radiopalmar quadrant of the fourth metacarpal. Dorsal III and dorsal II occupy the major areas of the third and second interspaces respectively and touch upon each other in an intramuscular septum which extends ulnarwards from the third metacarpal towards a septum lying between the flexor tendons of the third ray and the third lumbrical.

Palmar II borders on the adductor, just as dorsal I. It should be observed that at this level the adductor is not directly in contact with either the second or the third metacarpal, although it is quite possible that fibres originate from the deep palmar fascia. On tracing the interossei and adductor areas proximally, it becomes possible to follow their proximodistal development.

In the context of this paragraph, however, it seems to be appropriate to pinpoint only certain features: for instance, the very large size of the adductor at proximal levels and particularly its origin from the third metacarpal, including a few bundles from ligaments between the third and fourth metacarpals (Figs. 3.2 and 3.3).

Distoproximal screening establishes the origin of palmar III which is found on the palmar side of the fourth metacarpal as a few scattered bundles (Fig. 3.2). It is quite striking to see in Figure 3.3 that the space occupied by palmar IV and palmar III on the palmar side of the fifth and fourth metacarpals respectively, is occupied by the adductor in front of both the third and second metacarpals, whereas palmar II occupies the inner, or ulnar, aspect of the second metacarpal.

We have already made reference to the fairly extensive area of dorsal II. It is quite remarkable that the palmar tip of this area originates as part of the dorsal III area, which gradually becomes incorporated into dorsal II. This process of migration obviously requires the adductor to be released from the third metacarpal. This appears to happen distal to the passage of the deep palmar arch and it is easily seen that the passage of the radial artery over the second metacarpal takes place immediately distal to the origin of adductor bundles from ligaments anterior to the base of the second metacarpal

(Figs. 3.1 and 3.3). Distal to this passage we see the origin of an adductor bundle from the second metacarpal (Fig. 3.5) which is soon removed from the second metacarpal by the extending areas of dorsal I and palmar II (Fig. 3.9).

The passage of the deep palmar arch over the third metacarpal takes place over an adductor bundle covering this bone (Fig. 3.5), actually passing through a slit in the adductor. This adductor bundle separates the main area of dorsal II and a quadrangular-shaped area which eventually will be incorporated into the main dorsal II area. Once again it is obvious that this process requires the adductor bundle to be removed from the third metacarpal, and indeed this can be followed very neatly in Figures 3.5, 3.6, 3.7, 3.8 and 3.9. It is of particular importance to establish that this move of the accessory bundle is followed by the deep branch of the ulnar nerve passing between this small dorsal II bundle and the adductor thus gaining the deep space dorsal to the adductor.

Within the adductor area it has been possible to delimit the area representing the deep portion of the flexor pollicis brevis and the adductor proper (Fig. 3.1).

A topographic feature of some interest relates to the branch of the ulnar nerve to the flexor brevis. This branch is seen to pass between two adductor areas, areas which may be termed the oblique and the transverse portions of the muscle, to gain the flexor brevis; the latter is already spiralling around the tendon of the flexor pollicis longus (Fig. 3.8). The nerve runs over the free surface of the adductor below the first lumbrical and running behind the long flexor pollicis tendon comes close to the median nerve branches. It seems quite certain that we see here a form of Cannieu–Riche anastomosis.

In Figure 3.1, at the level of the proximal origin of the adductor, the most proximal tips of origin of the superficial bellies of the flexor pollicis brevis become apparent, one in the deepest layer of the flexor retinaculum just over the median nerve and the other in the superficial thenar compartment wall, just along the inner border of the abductor.

It is perhaps appropriate to observe here that the synovial cleft round the sublimis tendon of the fifth finger (which was seen to communicate with the ulnar bursa at carpal levels (Fig. 2.14) and which was only a tiny cleft in Figure 2.18) has widened considerably again at the levels just discussed.

At levels about those in Figures 2.21 and 3.2 the wall of this synovial cleft facing the ulnar bursa has become thinned out to such an extent that the presence of another passage can hardly be excluded.

In Figure 3.3 the distal end of the flexor retinaculum has been reached and the ulnar nerve and artery are seen in close apposition to the ulnar bursa while the latter is retracting from its sub-, inter- and supratendineal extensions.

The ulnar artery is just giving off a branch that will continue as the superficial palmar arch (Fig. 3.2) and another that will soon divide into deep and superficial branches. The deep branch is certain to anastomose with the deep palmar arch while the superficial one will be incorporated into the wall of the hypothenar area to continue its course with the nerve of the ulnar side of the little finger (Figs. 3.3 and 3.4). At these same levels the clefts around the superficial tendons II, III and IV attain their distal endpoints.

There is now a definite grouping of the flexor tendons of each finger although the lumbricals are still intimately related to the sleeves of the deep tendons. The median nerve is divided into its fascicles which diverge slightly from each other.

It would seem that we have now established the proximal base of the midhand which will enable us to evolve the columnar structure of the midhand in a logical manner.

It is well understood that the columns of the midhand, particularly hypothenar and thenar, extend well into the carpal area and therefore some overlap in the descriptions can hardly be avoided.

2. SEPARATE COLUMNS OF THE MIDHAND
The Thenar Compartment (*Series no. 1452*)

A zero-level is fixed where the abductor pollicis brevis appears in Figure 3.39. At this level the sheath of the flexor carpi radialis becomes attached to the tuberosity of the scaphoid bone. The abductor area occupies the space between the abductor longus and the flexor carpi radialis. Soon a second area appears, obviously originating from the flexor retinaculum. The two areas are separated from each other at their origin by the sheath of the flexor carpi radialis, but above the tuberosity of the trapezium they merge into one common area (Fig. 3.41).

A thin muscular sheet becomes visible about halfway over the trapezium and extends into the flexor retinaculum: the opponens pollicis. The opponens area can be easily identified as soon as the first metacarpal appears in the section (Fig. 3.43).

In the latter section the thenar space has become divided into two parts: an abductor area and an opponens area. The opponens area is increased greatly in thickness by the addition of fibres from the flexor retinaculum; the abductor area, divided into two more or less separate regions, gradually narrows and its ulnar border withdraws from the ulnar border of the thenar eminence (Figs. 3.43 and 3.46). Eventually it will be seen that the opponens area also contains the flexor brevis bundles. The extensive abductor area of Figure 3.43 becomes reduced to the thin area of Figures 3.46 and 3.47.

A muscular adductor area has become visible in the ligaments over the base of the capitate. This area enlarges over the ligaments covering the bases of the third and second metacarpals, which in their turn cover the tendon of the flexor carpi radialis, while the area widens in the niche between the first and second metacarpals (Figs. 3.45 and 3.46). This adductor area is divided into various areas according to the different directions of the fibres.

In Figure 3.46 there is still a well-defined abductor area and an opponens-flexor area, each of them being confined within one fascial space. An intramuscular septum separates the flexor-opponens area from the adductor area. In Figure 3.46 this septum can be traced from the crest of the first metacarpal (arrow) to the sheath of the flexor pollicis longus.

The septum is attached to the peritendineal layer of the flexor pollicis longus. It is, however, going to disappear and in its place a septum will develop within the adductor area, as a result of which a deep area becomes incorporated in the opponens-flexor area. From what can be seen in more proximal sections this deep flexor area arises between the area of the third metacarpal and the area which fills the niche between the first and second metacarpals. The new septum gradually becomes fully established (Fig. 3.47).

The opponens area can be defined as the area related to the first metacarpal. The flexor area is very extensive, passing on both sides of the opponens. The area derived from the adductor area can be determined without difficulty. Tendon formation is well on its way in the deep layer of the abductor. This typical picture persists in Figure 3.50 where the radial artery is seen to pass below the adductor, which has now lost contact with its area of origin.

An important re-grouping takes place at levels 547–631 where we are close to the metacarpophalangeal joint of the thumb. The opponens area has nearly come to an end. At its radial tip the abductor has formed a well-defined, pear-shaped tendon, which is in the process of joining with the hood of the extensor tendons (Fig. 3.52).

The wing of the extensor assembly begins to form in Figure 3.52 and comprises the abductor area (which can be recognized as such in proximal levels) with the superficial radial portion of the flexor, which has come between the opponens and the abductor proper (Figs. 3.47, 3.48 and 3.50). This portion can be clearly seen in Figure 3.52. If we follow this wing formation through the levels of Figure 3.52 to Figure 3.54, we see that the most radial portion of the superficial flexor component is gradually incorporated into the wing. From a comparison of these sections it also appears that the long extensor tendon is an independent rounded structure (Fig. 3.52). At this level the wing involves only the extensor brevis. In Figure 3.54 the extensor longus has become part of a layer which doubles the brevis layer, areolar tissue intervening between the two. A picture of the progress in the wing formation is given in Figure 3.60. The abductor proper is entirely tendinous and is oval-shaped in cross-section; the major part of the flexor division of the wing is also transformed into tendon fascicles. A superficial portion of the flexor appears to contribute to a pericapsular tendinous layer to which fibres of the deep portion also contribute.

The pericapsular tendon of the flexor brevis becomes a very impressive structure at levels where the radial metacarpophalangeal ligament is also visible. It is clear that the metacarpal origin of the latter takes place from a dorsally located tubercle. This implies that its course is an oblique one, like the directions of the same ligaments in the metacarpophalangeal joints of the fingers. Abduction movements allied with rotation are also likely to be feasible in the metacarpophalangeal joint of the thumb. The ulnar metacarpophalangeal ligament appears soon in subsequent sections. The ulnar wing is visible in Figure 3.60 and dorsally it divides over the two layers, the longus and the brevis layer, which are separated from each other by an areolar space. The ulnar wing continues into the fascial wall of the adductor compartment which is in close apposition to the capsule on the palmar aspect and into which adductor fascicles become inserted. Gradually, the extensor brevis tendon will fuse with the capsule and the lateral extension of its embedding layer ceases to maintain bilateral contact with the wing, with the result that an extensor

the abductor also finds its way into the laterobasal aspect of the phalangeal base.

Some of the adductor tendon fascicles pass into the sesamoid and some by-pass this area to reach the phalangeal base. The wing on this side is probably largely formed by palmar I and we have the impression that it remains a stronger layer than its counterpart on the radial side, although here too quite a few fibres delaminate to join capsular layers.

The Hypothenar Area (*Series no. 1452*)

The analysis of this area is begun proximally at the level where the deep fascia between the two flexors of the carpus divides to provide space ·for the fibres of the radial part of the abductor digiti V. At this same level the pisiform bone appears as a fibrous mass which is continuous with the extensor carpi ulnaris tendon sheath. The pisiform does not entirely invade the flexor carpi ulnaris tendon, because a considerable fibrous corona remains around the pisiform and on the ulnar side this fibrous tissue serves as the site of origin of the ulnar part of the abductor digiti V.

With the reduction in diameter of the pisiform area the two parts of the abductor digiti V join around the volar aspect of the pisiform (Fig. 3.39). In the groove where both parts of the muscle merge, a fibrous extension of the pisiform reinforces the fascia. This fibrous extension has been described as the pisiform skin anchor in Chapter 4 (Figs. 4.15 and 4.16).

Reinforcement of a deep fascial layer leads to the formation of the flexor retinaculum which runs below the ulnar nerve and vessels and continues as the ulnar wall of the flexor compartment and consequently at this level the ulnar nerve and vessels do not run in this compartment. Marked fibrous tracts originating from the pisiform area are seen in the superficial fascia covering the abductor digiti V. The pisiform area continues distally as two fibrous pillars, viz. the pisiform-hamate bundle and the ligamentum pisometacarpeum (Fig. 3.40). The marked pisiform skin anchor is also shown in this section. The first ligament becomes invaded by the hamulus ossis hamati, except for its medial part which runs in close apposition to the ulnar wall of the flexor compartment, so taking part eventually in the formation of the fibrous mass of origin of the palmar aponeurosis. The pisometacarpal bundle which is located in the deep fascial layer reinforces this layer as far as the hamate bone. The extensor carpi ulnaris tendon fuses now with its tendon sheath which also belongs to this deep fascia. A true insertion of the pisometacarpal ligament takes place into the base of the fifth metacarpal. The entire bundle does not deviate dorsally since one part runs directly distally while another moves medially and so skirts the ulnar aspect of the hamulus. The hamulus now extends volarwards as far as the ulnar nerve which crosses its volar tip (Fig. 3.41).

The radial border of the abductor digiti V gradually retreats towards the ulnar side just over the hamulus, as a result of which the radial branches of the ulnar nerve and vessels are no longer covered by the abductor digiti V but by the palmaris brevis only. At the same levels the hamulus ossis hamati gives origin to a muscle of the hypothenar complex in which two parts can be seen and which forms a wedge between what can be recognized now as the deep ulnar nerve and superficial branches.

Another muscular origin is found in the fascial duplicature lying immediately above the pisometacarpal bundle. This muscle, easily recognized as the deep part of the opponens digiti V, forms a wedge between the deep branches of the ulnar nerve and the pisometacarpal bundle which skirts the hamulus and so the deep ulnar nerve comes to lie between the two parts of the opponens digiti V (Fig. 3.42). The origins of these latter muscles are clear, viz. from the hamulus ossis hamati and from the volar and ulnar aspects of the ulnar flexor compartment wall of the flexor tunnel.

Distal to the hamulus, the radial part of the pisometacarpal bundle skirts the distal aspect of the hamulus radially. At this level and on both sides of the deep ulnar nerve new muscle bellies arise from the ulnar wall of the carpal tunnel and from the lateral aspect of the pisometacarpal bundle as the latter bundle proceeds medially below the floor of the flexor compartment.

The twin structures which arise from the wall of the flexor compartment on both sides of the deep ulnar nerve comprise palmar interosseus IV and a bundle which becomes incorporated in the opponens compartment (Fig. 3.44). As we will see later, one bundle of this area, though limited in size, becomes inserted into the volar plate. Tendon formation commences soon in the abductor area particularly close to the fascia at the inner upper corner of the compartment (Fig. 3.48). These tendons become surrounded by fascial envelopes derived from the compartment wall (Fig. 3.50).

The fascial roof of the hypothenar compartment is approached from the dorsal aspect by the dorsal intertendinous fascia in which we see the tendinous stretches of the extensors of the little finger. This fascial lamina now extends in the fascial layer between the abductor and the opponens, as a result of which the abductor tendon compartment becomes attached to the lateral side of this fibrofascial lamina (Fig. 3.51). While this process is going on two other phenomena attract our attention. Firstly there is the formation of a tendon in the opponens compartment and secondly the division of the volar intermuscular septum between palmar interosseus IV and opponens. The tendon formation in the opponens compartment involves the superficial layer. In the deep layer muscle fibres continue to be inserted into the metacarpal shaft (Fig. 3.51). Those fibres that converge upon the tendinous structure are inserted via this tendon into the retrocapsular region. At the same levels the medial wall of the abductor tendon compartment opens enabling this tendon to attain a true peri-articular position (Fig. 3.53). The intertendinous lamina which previously extended as a transverse lamina between the abductor and opponens compartments, now continues in its entirety lateral to the inner abductor tendon. Between this lamina transversa and the tendon we can see a bursa mucosa. In the capsular layers we see the metacarpo-glenoidal bundles with which the opponens tendon is merged. At retroarticular levels there are no longer any deep opponens fibres to be seen, as they are all inserted into the shaft of the metacarpal.

We do observe, however (Fig. 3.54), that there are still some muscular fibres in the area which are extending into the volar plate, but there is no indication whatsoever that the strong tendon which emerged from the opponens proceeds beyond the joint cleft. Hence only a minor portion of the opponens area behaves as a flexor digiti V brevis. We have still to determine the fate of the superficial division of the abductor in subsequent sections.

We will commence this final analysis with Figure 3.53 in which the inner abductor tendon has gained a juxtacapsular position. In the outer area a cluster of six or seven tendon fascicles is visible.

As a result of a gradual shift of the transverse lamina to the wall of the outer compartment the other tendon fascicles are guided into a juxtacapsular position. All abductor tendons are incorporated into the system of the external root of the volar plate (Fig. 3.55). The more distal development from this situation is found in Figures 3.57 and 3.58. The wing proper of the little finger merges with the external anchor of the volar plate, while both the wing and the volar plate provide fibres which extend into the skin of the latero-basal area. The phalangeal base absorbs the major part of this abductor external anchor system, with the exception of one tendon which will later form the wing of the extensor assembly.

The Hypothenar Area (*Series no. 1899*)

Because the hypothenar muscular column is rooted proximally in the carpal area, the proximal disposition of this area has been dealt with in the relative chapter.

The abductor digiti V finds its roots in the pisiform area (Fig. 2.11). The distal continuity of the flexor carpi ulnaris column, as far as the pisometacarpal ligament is concerned, passes towards the base of the fifth metacarpal; this results in space becoming available directly in front of the pisiform. In front of the pisiform and directly over the pisometacarpal ligament we see a strong fascial band passing from the hamulus to the metacarpal base. This ligament represents the proximal border of the deep opponens compartment (Fig. 2.16). At the level of the hamulus we come across two important phenomena, the course of the deep branch of the ulnar nerve and the origin of a muscular area arising from the tip of the hamulus. On approaching the hamulus the superficial division of the nerve maintains its level, while the deep branch passes into a deeper position. The reason for this can be found in the relative position of the hamulus and the pisiform for the hamulus lies not only distal to but also inwards from the pisiform.

It is quite obvious that the most lateral branch of the ulnar nerve (i.e. the deep branch) runs just lateral to the hamulus and thus reaches the deeper position. This deep branch passes over the rein forced proximal border of the deep opponens compartment and below a fibro-fascial bridge which extends from the hamulus to the abductor fascia. This bridge is soon to be replaced by a muscular area that will give rise to an additional abductor portion and also to the superficial opponens layer (Fig. 2.18); thus the deep branch of the ulnar nerve becomes situated between the two layers of the opponens. The division of the bundle arising from the tip of the hamulus into an additional abductor and the superficial opponens layer can be seen in Figures 2.17 to 2.21.

We will not here describe in detail the relationships of the medial aspect of the hypothenar as this has been dealt with extensively both in the section on the proximal midhand area and in the section on the hypothenar subcutaneous area. Suffice it to remark here that the passage of the ulnar nerve into the deep palmar space coincides with what may be called the displacement of the related intermuscular septum from the radial to the ulnar side of palmar IV.

At levels where the additional abductor area has already merged with the main abductor area (Figs. 3.4 and 3.5) tendon formation starts in the inner or juxtametacarpal muscular area. Quite soon (Fig. 3.6) six or seven small tendons become apparent, a phenomenon suggestive of a high structural and functional refinement within this muscle. On approaching the metacarpophalangeal joint one can see the particular way in which these tendons are led to the base of the phalanx (Figs. 3.8, 3.9 and 3.10). The extensor tendons of the little finger are embedded in a fascial layer which extends in an ulnar direction to the hypothenar compartment wall. We see that intramuscular septa arise as reinforcements of intramuscular fascias, just as we will see again in dorsal IV and II.

The septa formed in this way extend dorsal to the compartment wall where they readily become continuous with the transverse lamina of the extensor assembly of the little finger. In a palmar direction these septa serve as anchors for the abductor tendons in the volar plate of the joint. Disappearance of the juxtametacarpal compartment wall leads to each tendon attaining its juxtacapsular position. Following this procedure each tendon or group of tendons can be brought successively into the pericapsular position. It is obvious that the most superficial abductor tendon, being the last one to meet with the transverse lamina septum layer, is the only one to become a true wing tendon.

The transverse lamina in fact shifts over the roof of the compartment from medial to lateral (Figs. 3.11, 3.13 and 3.14). The superficial compartment, moreover, gives rise to a fairly strong pericapsular tendon that passes towards the laterobasal tubercle of the phalanx (Figs. 3.13, 3.14 and 3.15). It is only possible to distinguish a flexor digiti quinti brevis as part of the hypothenar on the basis of its origin from the hamulus. We have to recognize, however, that in this series this muscle gets entirely lost into the abductor: this point will be dealt with again in a microdissection of this area.

In summary the relations in this series can be easily surveyed. We can distinguish an opponens and an abductor muscle; the superficial opponens layer and an additional portion of the abductor arise proximally from the tip of the hamulus. The structural refinement within the abductor is most conspicuous.

The Hypothenar Area (*Series no. 1234*)

Further observations on the hypothenar area were made in *series no. 1234.* The most proximal origin of the abductor is found in the palmar fascia just above the ulnar nerve and vessels. Another portion of the abductor bundle emerges on the ulnar side of the pisiform area and while the pisiform disappears from the section, the two areas of the muscle come closer to each other and finally unite into one abductor area. The anterior aspect of the pisiform also serves as a site of origin of the abductor muscle. It is well worth noting how

far the muscle extends dorsally over the fascia lying between the
pisiform bone and the extensor carpi ulnaris tendon. Attention
should also be paid to the extension of the subcutaneous hypothenar
area.

At levels of the emergence of the hamulus in the piso-hamate
ligament, the picture is dominated by the division of the ulnar nerve
just above this bony prominence and the appearance of the deep
opponens as a ligamentous strand between the lateral side of the
hamulus and the base of the fifth metacarpal. Soon afterwards a
muscle bundle arises from the tip of the hamulus extending as an
opponens layer superficial to the deep ulnar nerve (Fig. 3.37). Just
distal to the hamulus some muscle strands arise from the ulnar flexor
compartment wall which do not immediately appear to be opponens
bundles because they display a fairly straight proximodistal course.
The two opponens layers move towards a common insertion into the
metacarpal shaft. A thin intermuscular septum separates the opponens
from palmar IV.

As soon as the opponens has become free from the ulnar flexor
compartment wall, the deep branch of the ulnar nerve gains the
deep palmar space and it becomes impossible to identify the bundles
from more proximal levels in the opponens area, which run more
longitudinally. While the opponens layer becomes increasingly
thin as a result of the insertion of its muscle bundles, tendon
formation in the abductor becomes more conspicuous and it seems
quite possible to distinguish an outer and inner muscular area.
Tendon formation is completed earlier in the inner area than in the
outer area. In fact when the inner tendon, or cluster, is approached in
the usual way by the transverse lamina system and led into pericapsular position, a muscular body of considerable extension can
still be seen in the outer area. Properly speaking there is no single
muscle fibre that could be designated as a flexor brevis. In the
opponens area no bundle extends beyond the metacarpophalangeal
joint. As for the abductor, its inner tendon, closely apposed to the
capsule, becomes absorbed with the latter into the phalangeal base.
The outer tendon of the abductor, initially on the outer side of the
transverse lamina, changes level with the latter so that it also obtains
a deep position. It transpires that this tendon merges into the outer
root of the volar plate. The transverse lamina remains slightly
adherent to this layer (Fig. 3.38).

Eventually the wing of the assembly detaches itself from the volar
structures. It cannot be made out precisely which part of the superficial portion of the abductor actually participates in the formation
of the wing, although a small part seems to do so. In fact the wing
has no properly reinforced volar border as in the other fingers.

Discussion of the Hypothenar Area

An adequate description of the arrangement of muscles in the
hypothenar does not seem to provide much difficulty. Tendon
formation in the abductor is extremely conspicuous and there is not
another muscle in the midhand which shows such a variety of
tendons and tendon fascicles. Most of these tendons become absorbed
into the base of the proximal phalanx. The tendons occur either in
small clusters or singly in a pericapsular position through a process

we will meet again in both dorsal and palmar interossei. This process involves (1) the formation of an intramuscular septum in contact with the medial and dorsal walls of the compartment; (2) the extension of the transverse lamina into such a septum and (3) the disappearance of the juxtacapsular compartment wall, so that the tendon enclosed in a juxtametacarpal compartment comes into a juxtacapsular position on the inner aspect of the transverse lamina; its path to the phalangeal base is quite straightforward.

The opponens arises in two layers from the hamulus and its distal continuity which is the ulnar flexor compartment wall. The layers pass on each side of the deep branch of the ulnar nerve.

In *series no. 1452* we saw that the superficial opponens layer contains one or two muscle bundles which can be traced distally downwards into the volar plate and, therefore, are to be considered as the flexor digiti V brevis.

In *series no. 1899* a fairly large area isolates itself from the superficial opponens area and gradually merges with the main abductor area. Although naturally some tendons emerging from this area run more volarwards than others, a flexor brevis can only be distinguished on the basis of its origin from the hamulus.

Finally in *series no. 1234* the opponens area does not contribute to the abductor and no flexor bundle can be distinguished in the former.

Palmar Interossei

Palmar interossei were also studied primarily in cross-sections of *series no. 1452*. The analysis will start at the basimetacarpal level and on viewing each cross-section the typical features of proximo-distal transformation will be noted.

The origin of palmar IV is found in a volar ligament inserted into the base of the fifth metacarpal and soon after palmar IV can be recognized as a rectangular area bordering the radiopalmar aspect of the fifth metacarpal between dorsal IV and the opponens digiti V. Palmar III is situated on the volar aspect of the fourth metacarpal, between (Fig. 3.48) dorsal IV and dorsal III, while palmar II appears to occupy the ulnar side of the second metacarpal.

The proximal roots of palmar IV and III can be clearly seen in Figures 3.44 and 3.45. In the former figure, palmar IV, associated with a bundle from the hamulus, appears as a twin-structure on both sides of the deep ulnar nerve. The second figure depicts the rectangle of palmar IV, while palmar III invests the palmar side of the fourth metacarpal.

While palmar IV and III are seen as large muscular areas, palmar II is more modest in extension on the cross-section, although quite soon (Fig. 3.54) the area of palmar II will extend considerably ulnarwards between dorsal II and the adductor. In the ulnar half of the section we already see a fascicle-type tendon formation of palmar IV and III.

Palmar IV

The cross-section picture of palmar IV (Fig. 3.53) is suggestive of a division of the muscle into an inner, juxtametacarpal part and an outer mass which fits over it as a cap. The tendon fascicles are visible in the inner part and also to some extent in an intramuscular cleft.

The convergence of muscular fibres on the tendon mass proceeds in such a way that the tendon is displaced towards the joint while still covered by a muscular mass.

The process of tendon formation can be followed easily in subsequent sections. The fascicle-type arrangement within the muscle, already seen in Figure 3.53, continues to be quite evident. In subsequent sections (Figs. 3.58 and 3.59) several conspicuous features attract our attention.

Some grouping or clustering in tendon fascicles seems to take place so that both a central mass and a dorsal accessory tendon can be seen. Juxtacapsular muscle bundles do not join the central tendon; they are seen instead to form a tendinous lamina that will become inserted into the volar plate of the joint (Fig. 3.61). The resulting inner tendinous layer joins with the distal border of the transverse lamina proper, so that the inner tendon layer will henceforth occupy this stratum (Figs. 3.61, 3.63 and 3.64).

It can be seen in the latter figure that the dorsal tendon contributes considerably to this inner tendon layer. The anchoring system of palmar IV does not entirely disappear in the volar plate. The main palmar tendon will join the inner layer of Figure 3.64, so that, after the transverse lamina has contacted the tip of the tendon, a club-shaped wing results (Fig. 3.65). We have observed that the tendon disburses some fibres from the wing into pericapsular strata just as will be seen to occur in palmar III. These pericapsular layers are continuous with the infratendineal layers at more proximal levels. The infratendinous fascia blends with the capsule and becomes inserted into periosteal layers (Landsmeer, 1955).

In this series we see that the infratendinous layer changes level: instead of continuing into the pericapsular strata it merges with the wing of the extensor assembly, which is the reason for its becoming suspended from the base of the phalanx (Fig. 3.65). A disbursement of fibres from the tendon appears to continue, as is seen in figures like 3.67, 3.69 and 3.71; the disbursed fibres join pericapsular layers.

The fourth lumbrical begins to converge its fibres towards the upper corner of its compartment where they come in close contact with the volar plate. As seen in Figure 3.69 a portion of the lumbrical becomes inserted into the capsule. Beyond the distal border of the transverse intermetacarpal ligament the majority of lumbrical fibres joins the wing of the extensor assembly. Some small fascicles join pericapsular layers (Fig. 3.74).

Palmar III

Tendon formation in palmar III becomes visible at the level of Figure 3.58. Tendon fascicles are grouped in the form of an *H*. Gradually the tendon moves closer to the bone as a result of muscle bundles in this area joining the tendon system. Tendon formation is somewhat simpler here than in palmar IV. At the level of Figure 3.66 the tendon in palmar III has already moved fairly close to the bone. Eventually a picture develops that is fairly similar to that encountered in palmar IV. After the insertion of a few muscle bundles into the juxtametacarpal compartment wall, we see a juxtametacarpal tendon which collects muscle fibres from the dorsal tip of the muscle, just as occurs in palmar IV. This tendon in palmar IV was seen to replace the transverse lamina. In palmar III the transverse lamina persists and the inner tendon runs along its outer aspect (Fig. 3.77). Gradually the tendon fascicles come close to the juxtametacarpal compartment wall. By collecting the fibres on its inner side the tendon is transformed into a flat band, lying close to the transverse lamina. We see the insertion of a few tiny muscle bundles into the juxtametacarpal compartment wall, the latter being identical to the transverse lamina. Furthermore it seems that fibres from the outer muscular area skirt the volar tip of the tendon and are also inserted into the transverse lamina. By this process the transverse lamina breaks away from the transverse intermetacarpal ligament so that a picture results like that in Figure 3.79 or Figure 3.80.

It is obvious that it requires only one more step to incorporate the tendon into the transverse lamina, so enabling a proper wing to be formed. As Figure 3.83 shows, while the transverse lamina ceases to exist on the volar aspect its dorsal portion shifts to the interosseous tendon so that a continuous wing results. The insertion of the lumbrical into this wing follows, distal to the transverse intermetacarpal ligament. The insertion, or attachments, of the lumbrical into the volar plate are far less impressive than those of lumbrical IV.

Palmar II

In the general introduction mention has been made already of the proximal origin of palmar II from the ulnar aspect of the second metacarpal. The area of this muscle at proximal levels is quadrangular or trapezoidal and it gradually expands below the area of dorsal II (Figs. 3.48 and 3.54). Tendon formation in this muscle proceeds from a flat tendon layer lying in the sagittal plane of the hand (Figs. 3.60 and 3.72). The fascicles composing the plate grow steadily so that the whole plate becomes thicker. More tiny tendon fascicles become apparent, growing like a palmar tail from the main tendon. This situation remains stable for some time, the main dorsal tendon growing in thickness while the palmar fascicles become more marked and arrange themselves in a frontal plane (Fig. 3.77). Gradually a very typical cross-section results (Fig. 3.84), viz. one which shows a main dorsal tendon, in which the separate fascicles are still distinct and the palmar fascicles seem to cluster into two groups. These palmar fascicles eventually join to form one tendon, so that the situation is now (Fig. 3.88) that two tendons emerge from the muscle body, a dorsal and a palmar. These two tendons, which have become rounded in the meantime, derive fibres from the respective areas of the muscle so that two solid cords eventually dominate the cross-section of palmar II, the dorsal one remaining somewhat thicker than the palmar one (Fig. 3.89).

A picture as in Figure 3.91 is seen, in which a fascia-like intramuscular septum has developed between the tendons, strongly suggesting some resemblance between this palmar interosseus development and dorsal interosseus II or IV. The spatial disposition within the muscle and in the formation of the tendons seem to be distinctly more simple than in the dorsal interossei.

The intramuscular septum is seen to gain in importance; the juxtametacarpal fascicle wall disappears so that the dorsal tendon gradually moves into its pericapsular position (Figs. 3.92 and 3.94) and is anchored to the volar plate through the fascial layers around it. The transverse lamina extends into the intramuscular septum so that the tendons become suspended from this layer, the dorsal tendon lying in a deeper position than the palmar one. In a picture such as Figure 3.94 the cross-section view of palmar II closely resembles that of the tendon formation of dorsal III. The wing of the extensor assembly has been formed and no marked changes are taking place, as a result of which it appears that palmar II produces a multi-fasciculate wing tendon anchored to the volar plate of the meta-carpophalangeal joint with fibrofascial extensions. As subsequent sections show (Figs. 3.95, 3.97 and 3.100) the entire tendon complex is transformed into the wing of the extensor assembly. The tendon complex and also the wing remain basically free of the anchoring system of the volar plate and tendon sheath, in contrast to the situation in dorsal III.

Summary Palmar Interossei (series no. 1452)

Summarizing the situation in the palmar interossei of this series it can be concluded that despite some definite similarities certain conspicuous differences are obvious. Palmar II turns out to be the most complicated of this series. The double tendon in the muscle is quite characteristic. The intramuscular septum and the final formation of a multifasciculate wing tendon is strongly reminiscent of the situation in dorsal III. Palmar III seems to represent the most simply structured of all the palmar interossei. Apart from attachments into the volar plate, one tendon plate becomes transformed into the radial wing of the fourth finger. Although in palmar IV the final result of its insertion is very similar to that for palmar III, it should be noted that in palmar IV the intramuscular arrangement is more complex than in palmar III and its tendon is markedly more fasciculated than that of palmar III. Thus it seems to be that palmar II is the most refined of the palmar interossei, then comes palmar IV and then palmar III.

We used a second series to try to verify the constitution of the palmar interossei, *series no. 1899*.

The proximal origin in *series no. 1899* has already been dealt with in the general introduction and we have established a close similarity between the two *series 1899* and *1452*. Therefore, we will pass now to levels at which tendon formation is well on its way; and in Figure 3.16 we clearly see tendon fascicles in palmar II, the *H*-shaped disposition in palmar III and, in palmar IV, a marked tendon complex in the dorsal area with tiny fascicles in the palmar portion of the muscle.

Palmar IV

In the latter muscle (Figs. 3.17 and 3.19) the main dorsal tendon draws closer to the juxtametacarpal compartment wall and after the disappearance of this wall the main dorsal tendon of the muscle comes to its pericapsular position (Fig. 3.22). Moreover, as seen in this picture, this tendon becomes firmly anchored to the volar plate of the joint. This anchorage is effected by some of the peripheral fascicles of the main tendon, so that the core of the tendon runs freely along the ligaments of the joint. At the same time the superficial tendon runs on the outer side of the anchoring fascicles (Fig. 3.23). The deep fascicle becomes incorporated in the pericapsular system so that it becomes suspended from the tubercle of the metacarpal head. This situation virtually predicts the incorporation of the deep tendon into the capsular system and its eventual insertion into the phalangeal base. The anchoring fascicles eventually join the deep tendon (Figs. 3.25, 3.26, 3.27 and 3.29). The superficial or palmar tendon becomes part of the infratendinous fascia for a while, a situation we found in the previous series. This tendon eventually becomes one layer by joining with the extensor tendon so that a true wing of the extensor assembly is formed (Figs. 3.29 and 3.30).

Palmar III

In palmar III the tendon fascicles seem to concentrate more or less into one central cluster (Fig. 3.28). Gradually the tendon moves close to the joint and becomes situated deep in the ulno-palmar niche of the compartment (Fig. 3.30). Then the tendon extends dorsally along the compartment wall, representing there the deep layer of a triangular shaped muscle area (Fig. 3.32).

As is seen in Figure 3.34 the transverse lamina obtains a free palmar border even before the tendon of palmar III becomes incorporated into it. The latter process takes place in a peculiar way as can be observed in Figure 3.35. The transverse lamina extends around the wing tendon fascicles forming a kind of sling around them, so establishing a new free palmar border of the wing.

Palmar II

The formation of two tendons in palmar II is just as conspicuous here as it is in *series no. 1452* (Figs. 3.27 and 3.30). Of the two the palmar tendon is definitely more voluminous than the dorsal one. The dorsal tendon draws closer to the juxtametacarpal compartment wall and because of the disappearance of this wall and the extension of the transverse lamina between the two tendons, the dorsal tendon comes to lie in a pericapsular position (Fig. 3.32). It is also evident in this picture that the now pericapsularly placed tendon is much smaller than the palmar one, which continues to run lateral to the compartment wall. The pericapsular tendon becomes gradually lost by absorption into the base of the phalanx. The palmar tendon is finally attached to the transverse lamina and thus forms a wing of the extensor assembly (Figs. 3.34, 3.35 and 3.36).

Summary Palmar Interossei (series no. 1899)

Summarizing this series we find that the internal arrangement of both palmar IV and palmar II are more complicated and refined than that of palmar III. In palmar IV the picture shows two tendons emerging from the muscle, while further tendinous anchors to the transverse intermetacarpal ligament are found. A pericapsular tendon becomes suspended from the metacarpal head and this eventually becomes inserted into the phalangeal base. The palmar tendon becomes a wing tendon. A similar situation prevails in palmar II, where the dorsal tendon also obtains a pericapsular position and becomes lost within this system. The major palmar tendon proceeds distally as a wing tendon. Palmar III is somewhat simpler in texture and internal arrangement. A tendon emerges from this muscle which constitutes the radial wing of the assembly of the fourth finger.

General Discussion of Palmar Interossei

Comparison of the two series shows that some consistency exists in the internal structure of the various muscles and their insertion pattern.

Series no. 1899 showed a major dorsal tendon and a minor palmar one for palmar IV. The dorsal tendon found a phalangeal insertion and the palmar tendon formed the wing.

In *series no. 1452* the division of the tendon mass into dorsal and palmar components was distinctly less conspicuous than in *series no. 1899*. We could see, however, that tendinous fascicles from the dorsal area provided a strong anchorage for the tendon into the transverse intermetacarpal ligament. In *series no. 1452* palmar IV resembles palmar III to some extent, although tendon formation in the latter seems to be based on a much more simple internal arrangement of the muscle. Palmar III figured in both series as the simplest of the three. Tendon formation did not seem to be so complicated, in both series a single tendon ran along the transverse lamina and continued into the radial wing of the ring finger.

The internal arrangement of palmar II is fairly complicated giving rise to dorsal and palmar tendons. In *series no. 1452* the tendons eventually all assembled to form the ulnar wing, thereby forming the multifasciculate tendon as we know it from dorsal III. *Series no. 1899* showed a double insertion, of which the dorsal tendon passed into the phalangeal base and the palmar one continued as the wing.

General Summary of Palmar Interossei

The analysis of the palmar interossei has revealed a basic difference among the muscles of this group in which we have included palmar II, III and IV: palmar I having been described in the paragraph on the thenar musculature. Tendon formations in palmar II and IV may entail some variation in the insertion of these interossei. The major point about these interossei seems to be that each may form more than one tendon, which is particularly conspicuous for palmar II in both series. In one series (*no. 1452*) palmar II behaved as if it were a regular dorsal III, the two tendons being suspended from the transverse lamina, resulting in a fairly complicated tendon. In *series no. 1899* the dorsal tendon of palmar II was inserted into the phalangeal base in close apposition to the capsule. The palmar tendon was transformed into the wing. In palmar IV we saw the formation of a double tendon in *series no. 1899*, the dorsal one of which eventually became inserted into the phalangeal base, while the palmar or superficial one continued into the wing of the little finger. In *series no. 1452* the tendon complex passed largely into the wing, while anchorage into the volar plate was a marked phenomenon. In palmar III an *H*-like tendon was found at proximal levels. Tendon formation is definitely simpler in this muscle than in either palmar II or palmar IV; in both series the tendon continued into the wing of the assembly.

Dorsal Interossei

In an earlier study we presented an extensive report on the internal structural arrangement of dorsal IV (Landsmeer, 1965). This analysis yielded some quite interesting results about tendon formation and in particular about the role of this muscle in the constitution of the metacarpophalangeal area. The arrangement in the metacarpophalangeal area and the insertion pattern of the interosseus are closely related to each other.

It soon turned out that the arrangement found in dorsal IV does not apply rigorously to the other dorsal interossei. The internal arrangement of dorsal II is closest to dorsal IV. Salsbury (1937) found a close similarity in the insertion pattern of these muscles.

Dorsal III, although it displays the basic features of a dorsal interosseus just as dorsal II, behaves differently in the metacarpophalangeal region which results in a different form of insertion. Dorsal I is in a fairly unique position with regard to size and insertion and it is, in a way, the most simple of all the dorsal interossei.

Dorsal IV

We now present a brief analysis of dorsal IV, based on earlier work. The close resemblance between dorsal II and dorsal IV facilitates the analysis and as dorsal II and dorsal III belong to the same ray it is easy to follow these muscles in the same cross-sections simultaneously.

In our previous analysis of dorsal IV we made use of *series no. 1452* and checked the results against other series, both transverse and frontal. One of the control series chosen was *series no. 1899* which also has served as the key-series for both the carpal area and the base of the midhand. A second control used was *series no. 1279*, which is a transverse section of the third ray only, and thus covered only dorsal II and dorsal III. Finally some typical cross-sections of dorsal IV in *series no. 1900* have been included. We propose to follow this order again so that we turn now to *series no. 1452* in Figure 3.49 in which is shown a proximal level of the fourth intermetacarpal space.

At these proximal levels we may distinguish basically two main muscle bellies, radial and ulnar, as well as a deep additional belly which becomes apparent in the ulnar niche at the attachment of the intramuscular septum between palmar III and dorsal IV in metacarpal IV. This portion of the muscle gradually encroaches upon this septum in a palmar direction. A fascicle-type tendon formation takes place in the intramuscular cleft between the main bellies of the muscle. The main radial belly of the muscle extends further palmarwards than the ulnar belly so that the cleft butts against the septum between dorsal IV and palmar IV. Concentration of muscle fibres into the tendinous fascicles leads to a considerable thinning of the volar portion of the main area. The space thus gained is occupied by a considerable extension of the deep additional radial belly, whereas on the dorsal aspect of the muscle contributions still seem to be given to the main areas from the fourth and fifth metacarpals (Fig. 3.53). Soon we can see that tendon fascicles in the dorsal portion fuse into one main central tendon, a conspicuous structure (Fig. 3.56) which continues to collect muscle bundles. This process proceeds in a peculiar fashion as can be seen in Figures 3.59, 3.61 and 3.64. It is quite clear that the central tendon obtains fibres from the radiodorsal area of the muscle as a whole, but that the extreme radiodorsal quadrant of this area becomes transformed into two tiny juxtametacarpal tendons instead of sending its fibres to the central tendon. It is also apparent that the true transverse fibres and the fibres approaching the tendon from the dorsal aspect constitute a tendinous whorl. The outermost branch of this whorl (Fig. 3.64) can soon be seen to extend as an intramuscular septum between the radiodorsal area and the rest of the muscle.

We should ascertain first that the dorsal or main tendon has moved closer to the fourth metacarpal through this process of tendon formation. Passing the origin of the interossei and approaching close to the metacarpophalangeal region it is obvious that a juxtametacarpal fascia or compartment wall will present. This situation anticipates that in which the intramuscular septum, derived from the central tendon, blends with the juxtametacarpal compartment wall in a palmar direction, while its dorsal extension leads to contact with the dorsal compartment wall.

As soon as the compartment wall of the dorsal juxtametacarpal quadrant vanishes the following relationship is effected: the dorsal main tendon gains a juxtacapsular position and the way is now open for the formation of a transverse lamina between the extensor tendon and the palmar capsule. The transverse lamina is in fact the distal continuity of the intramuscular septum (Figs. 3.66, 3.67 and 3.69).

As can be seen in Figure 3.61, some of the tendon fascicles and an important muscle area are not involved in the formation of the dorsal main tendon.

Some tendon fascicles have emerged from what we have described as the tail of the main two-bellied part of the muscle. Earlier we distinguished an intermediate tendon and a volar tendon among these tendon fascicles. The intermediate tendon, which collected fibres from more proximal levels, is left for quite some distance without further addition of muscle fibres. The volar tendon itself is composed of various fascicles and will obtain fibres from part of the additional radial belly. The fibres of this part of the additional radial belly run mainly transversely and are located just palmar to the main radial belly (Fig. 3.64). The remaining part of the additional radial belly contributes to the main volar tendon and to a flat tendinous lamina developing on the ulnar side of the main volar tendon. This lamina obtains also fibres from the ulnodorsal portion of the muscle. This ulnar tendinous lamina now comes in contact with the intermediate tendon passing over the main volar tendon. In this way a sling is formed around the main volar tendon (Figs. 3.64, 3.67 and 3.69). This tendinous sling is derived from the muscle itself and becomes anchored to the transverse intermetacarpal ligament (Figs. 3.69, 3.71 and 3.72) so holding the main volar tendon in a well-defined position with respect to the head of the metacarpal.

Later we see that the dorsal tendon becomes virtually incorporated in pericapsular layers as it lies in its pericapsular position. In this situation both the tendon and the ligaments of the joint become invaded by the base of the phalanx so that a true phalangeal insertion is established. At this point we should refer to the intimate relationship between the anchoring interosseous tendon and the external anchor of the volar plate (Fig. 3.76), a point which will be described further in Chapter IV.

Let us now look more closely at what is happening to the main palmar tendon. It is already understood that this tendon will become the tendon forming the extensor assembly and so is a true wing tendon. Figures 3.69 and 3.71 show that this tendon is located strictly lateral to the transverse lamina. In Figure 3.72 this layer has obtained a distal free border on its palmar aspect, while the remaining transverse lamina contacts the inner part of the tendinous loop, so re-establishing its continuity with the transverse intermetacarpal ligament. Further distally this continuity is broken again causing the transverse lamina to move to the layer of the main palmar tendon. A continuity between transverse lamina and this tendon requires that the tendon should fuse with the top of the tendinous loop (Fig. 3.74). Remarkably enough the inner part of the loop now delaminates from the wing system to gain a pericapsular position covering the phalangeal tendon. The outer part of the loop becomes a fascial covering of the wing tendon. Figure 3.74 shows this layer to continue in a palmar direction remaining fairly tendinous and merging into the fibrofascial systems around vessels and nerves and the lumbrical muscle.

At levels of the phalangeal base the layer covering the phalangeal tendons is still recognizable as a layer extending from the tendon sheath and volar plate in a dorsal direction (Figs. 3.76 and 3.81). It will be clear from these sections that the phalangeal base absorbs the dorsal tendon which is covered by the inner part of the sling, while the main palmar tendon extends distally as the wing of the assembly. It is clear from the foregoing that the basic division of a dorsal interosseus into phalangeal and wing tendons is effected by a most refined intramuscular arrangement.

We checked a few other series to verify these findings. Because the cross-section views of dorsal IV are so characteristic, it will suffice to present here only a few of the cross-sections in each case.

In Figure 3.3 (*series no. 1899*) we see the typical cross-section of a dorsal interosseus. The perforating artery is just passing through the intramuscular cleft. At these proximal levels this series does not permit us to delineate precisely the dorsal bellies from the palmar radial belly. Tendon formation emerges in the intramuscular cleft and quite soon (Fig. 3.10) a conspicuous formation becomes apparent in the dorsal portion of the main bellies; this is followed soon by an additional tail-like cluster in the palmar portion of the main bellies (Fig. 3.13). In this section it is quite possible to distinguish the palmar radial belly from the remainder of the muscle. In this same figure there is some indication of early whorling within the dorsal tendon while a dorsoradial quadrant, that will not become involved in the main dorsal tendon, can also be distinguished. A few sections further on (Fig. 3.15) the cross-section is very characteristic of a fourth dorsal interosseus, the main features being spiralling in the dorsal tendon, a segregation of a dorsoradial quadrant and further tendon formation in the ulnodorsal corner of the palmar portion of the muscle. It can be clearly seen that both the main dorsal tendon and tendons in the palmar area collect transverse fibres. Formation of an intramuscular septum can be followed in Figures 3.17 and 3.19. It seems quite certain that this septum represents the distal continuity of the transverse arm of the whorl and of the muscle lamina just ulnar to the main dorsal tendon. This septum merges into or replaces the juxtacapsular compartment wall which also becomes reinforced by a tiny tendon from the upper dorsoradial quadrant. The main dorsal tendon soon moves into a juxtacapsular position (Figs. 3.21 and 3.22).

A transverse lamina will extend now towards the roof of the compartment and will become continuous with the intramuscular septum. The juxtacapsular tendon gradually becomes entirely incorporated in the pericapsular lamina.

Figure 3.26 shows that a kind of delamination has occurred in the dorsal tendon so that one part of the tendon serves as a covering layer for the other. The palmar tendon complex, situated on the outer side of the transverse lamina, becomes elongated and tends to become anchored to the transverse intermetacarpal ligament. Figure 3.28 shows that it seems to be the most dorsal tendon of the palmar system which extends on both sides of the palmar one, thus forming a sling for the latter.

This situation becomes more marked in subsequent sections, and in Figure 3.29 we can establish an anchorage of the palmar tendon to the transverse intermetacarpal ligament and an extension through this ligament into the palmar area, notably around the tendon sheath. Again, further distally the superficial tendon becomes suspended from the transverse lamina so forming a true wing (Fig. 3.30).

It is very striking that the process of wing formation occurs in this series in exactly the same way as in *series no. 1452*. It can be noticed directly in Figures 3.30, 3.31 and 3.33 that an inner layer of the tendon delaminates from the main tendon and joins the phalangeal tendon; hence the wing proper represents the main palmar tendon.

Just a few sections are shown here of a third series (*no. 1900*) in which dorsal IV was investigated.

Figure 3.101 presents another example of an intramuscular septum continuing into the juxtametacarpal compartment wall. The dorsal tendon moves nearly into a juxtacapsular position. In Figure 3.102 this same tendon extends into the volar plate. Notice the thin juxtacapsular twin tendon on its inner side. In Figure 3.103 the dorsal tendon has gained a juxtacapsular position; it is seen as a doubled structure which blends with the infratendinous fascia dorsally and fuses with the system of volar plate and tendon sheath palmarwards. The transverse lamina continues into the inner part of the sling that holds the future wing tendon.

Dorsal II

In the same *series no. 1452* we assessed tendon formation in dorsal II and found it to be very similar to the pattern of dorsal IV. As dorsal III will be seen to be basically different from these two, it will be particularly instructive to study dorsal II and III simultaneously. First, however, we will discuss these muscles separately.

In *series no. 1452* dorsal II presents as a large area which at a proximal level (Fig. 3.62) shows a striking resemblance to dorsal IV (cf. Fig. 3.53). A main dorsal area is composed of a radial and an ulnar belly, the latter forming the tip of the tail of this area. A deep portion is also added to the muscle, originating from the radiopalmar aspect of the third metacarpal and from the intramuscular septum attached to this bone. It is obvious that dorsal II is the mirror-image of dorsal IV.

Tendon formation becomes more and more marked and in Figure 3.66 a cluster of tendon fascicles can be seen in the dorsal part of the muscle and also a tail of fascicles in the palmar portion of the main two-bellied part of the muscle. A deep palmar portion has already considerable size. The dorsal cluster tends to concentrate into one solid tendon (Fig. 3.80). Soon an intramuscular septum emerges, just as in dorsal IV, by virtue of the elongation of the outermost layer of the dorsal tendon in both palmar and dorsal directions. A picture results like that seen in Figure 3.84. Although the constellation is perhaps not as sharply marked as that of dorsal IV in Figure 3.64, the picture is basically identical. It is certainly most striking that the juxtametacarpal twin tendon of dorsal IV is present as well, although at this point the two have obviously fused with each other.

The picture seen in Figure 3.84 seems somewhat complicated by the fact that in it the intermediate tendon is fused with the layer that will become the intramuscular septum. In further sections this tendon behaves as an intramuscular septum as it joins the true septum also in a dorsal direction (Fig. 3.89).

It is not surprising, therefore, that the formation of a tendinous loop over the main tendon in the palmar area is far less marked than in dorsal IV. We note that in dorsal IV the tendinous loop over the palmar tendon was derived to a great extent from the intermediate tendon. Figure 3.89 shows clearly an extraordinarily thick septum in dorsal II into which the transverse lamina has already, at least partly, found its continuity. Disappearance of the juxtametacarpal compartment wall will place the dorsal tendon in a juxtacapsular position. On the outer side of the transverse lamina the palmar tendon lies directly against the transverse lamina, only a thin fascia-like band intervening. It is quite interesting to compare this picture with the corresponding section of dorsal IV (Fig. 3.67) to observe the strong tendon on the inner side of the palmar tendon in the latter. This strong tendon was derived from the intermediate tendon. Actually in this specimen a true anchorage of the palmar tendon by means of a tendinous loop does not seem to be present. As we mentioned, however, there are fascial structures that hold the tendon in this position (Fig. 3.94). The invasion of the phalangeal tendon by the base of the phalanx is imminent in Figure 3.98. In this picture it is interesting to observe the blending of this tendon of the interosseus with the suspension apparatus of the tendon sheath at metacarpo-phalangeal level; a situation which seems even more marked in Figure 3.99.

Dorsal III

The internal structure of this muscle develops distally on the proximal pattern of a dorsal interosseus. In this muscle also we see a main dorsal tendon, built up of various fascicles and a palmar tendon composed of different fascicles (Fig. 3.65). This muscle differs, however, from dorsal II and dorsal IV in the following respects: no spiralling of the dorsal tendon occurs; there is absence of the juxtametacarpal twin tendons; there is no formation of an intramuscular septum and therefore the transverse lamina continues directly into the juxtameta-carpal compartment wall. As for the last point, it is clear that this arrangement means that the entire tendon system of the muscle becomes located on the outer surface of the transverse lamina and that a phalangeal tendon is likely to be absent, all the tendon fascicles sharing in the formation of a wing to the extensor assembly.

We will now resume the proximodistal analysis starting from the level at which the cross-section view resembles that of dorsal IV. In Figure 3.65 we can distinguish the main dorsal tendon composed of different fascicles and the tail-like volar tendon which obtains fibres from the radial main belly. In a picture like Figure 3.75 this process is seen to be nearly accomplished. The dorsal main tendon is a round cord, while the volar tendon is still a tail-like structure on cross-section. Gradually a round major palmar tendon becomes apparent, in close apposition to the fascicles of the dorsal tendon (Fig. 3.77). The remainder of the muscle fascicles of this area converges on a minor palmar tendon. A Figure such as 3.78 clearly shows the absence of the juxtametacarpal tendons which are so typical of dorsal IV and of dorsal II. Furthermore, in this section tendon fascicles have appeared in the palmar radial portion of the muscle. These fascicles will soon join the palmar tendon originating at more proximal levels. In the meantime, in the dorsal tendon, now in juxtametacarpal position, the fascicles have arranged themselves in such a way that a kind of hilum in the cross-section is formed; from this hilum, fibres leave the tendon complex in a palmar direction (Fig. 3.79) and extend further in the same direction eventually anchoring the dorsal tendon to the transverse intermetacarpal ligament (Fig. 3.82). This anchorage is soon followed by an anchoring of the lateral bundle of the dorsal tendon (Figs. 3.83 and 3.84), while the juxtametacarpal bundle now replaces the juxtametacarpal compartment wall. Accepted that the transverse lamina is placed in line with this wall, the situation is now such that the transverse lamina and the innermost tendon fascicle are in alignment with one another. More tendon fascicles have emerged in the palmar area of the muscle. The situation allows us to distinguish a major and a minor palmar tendon (Fig. 3.80). The minor tendon soon gains in importance (Fig. 3.82), then no longer differs much in size while an additional bundle provides an anchorage for the palmar tendon complex to the palmar ligaments (Figs. 3.84 and 3.85). The major palmar tendon maintains a definite individuality and finds its way into the wing of the assembly. The anchorages being passed, the tendon complex becomes suspended from the transverse lamina (Fig. 3.86) and gradually the interosseous fibres fan out to form the fibrous wing of the assembly (Figs. 3.87, 3.89, 3.90, 3.93 and 3.96).

We are able to confirm the constitution of both dorsal II and dorsal III in *series no. 1899*, and Figure 3.32 provides a fine example of the characteristic arrangement in both muscles. In dorsal II the distinct dorsal tendon surrounded by a semicircular layer is quite a conspicuous feature and it will be transformed into the intramuscular septum. In the dorsoradial area, tendon formation is very different from that observed in dorsal IV since the tendons in the centre of the muscle area are absent. The arrangement of dorsal III is quite characteristic, with the anchorage of the multifasciculate dorsal tendon to the volar plate and the palmar tendons running freely along this main tendon complex.

Figure 3.34 shows that in dorsal III the transverse lamina passes through the muscle so that the main dorsal tendon comes into a juxtacapsular position, with the palmar tendon running along its outer side.

In dorsal II the main dorsal tendon is already in a close pericapsular position and the palmar area of this muscle resembles a palmar interosseus. Further distally the transverse lamina in dorsal III has incorporated both the tendons visible in Figure 3.34 so that the situation develops into that shown in Figure 3.35. In dorsal II the dorsal tendon moves into a juxtacapsular position and eventually becomes inserted into the phalangeal base. The palmar complex becomes joined with the second lumbrical suspended from the transverse lamina and thus forms the wing of the assembly on the radial side of the middle finger.

We can verify the tendon formation of both dorsal II and III in *series no. 1279*, in Chapter 5 of this book on the fibrous constitution of the finger, where Figures 5.53, 5.52, 5.51, 5.50, 5.48 and 5.35 provide ample evidence of the key-features of both these muscles. In dorsal II we see the division of the muscle by the transverse lamina formed from the continuity of an intramuscular septum. A phalangeal tendon is situated deep to this layer and the eventual wing tendon on its outside aspect. In contrast to this in dorsal III we see the transverse lamina continuing into the juxtametacarpal compartment wall. Conspicuous in both muscles are the anchorages of the respective tendons to the volar plate (Figs. 5.52, 5.51, 5.50 and 5.49). The fascicle-type constitution of the tendon complex of dorsal III is also a marked phenomenon in this series. Just as in *series no. 1452* the main dorsal tendon of dorsal III displays a form of hilum from which fibres extend in a palmar direction (Fig. 5.49). The transverse lamina merges with this tendon layer so that the tendon is divided into two by the transverse lamina and its continuity. The phalangeal tendon of dorsal II that is firmly anchored to the palmar pad becomes gradually suspended from the dorsolateral tubercle at the phalangeal base (Fig. 5.47).

In view of the fact that the tendons of both dorsal II and III contribute to the volar plate (including the metacarpophalangeal tendon sheath) it is not surprising that the outer root of the suspension system of the tendon sheath and the phalangeal tendon of dorsal II should merge into each other (Fig. 5.48). In contrast to this arrangement, on the ulnar side an anchoring layer of the tendon sheath and volar plate complex obviously keeps entirely clear of the wing tendon complex of dorsal III (Fig. 5.45). The final formation of the wings of the assembly of the middle finger can be followed in Figure 5.43 and subsequent sections. The multifasciculate structure of the tendon and the wing of dorsal III is most conspicuous. On the radial side the wing is reinforced by a lumbrical muscle.

Dorsal I

In an earlier analysis of dorsal I, based on dissections (Landsmeer, 1955) it was clear that the inner structure of this muscle is quite easily determined; it is also a very large muscle which makes a serial microscopic analysis superfluous. We therefore chose a few sections only in which to demonstrate the tendon formation.

In Figure 3.21 tendon fascicles are seen to emerge in the intramuscular cleft and the extension of the muscle in a palmar direction is quite conspicuous. A similar pattern prevails in Figure 3.24. To some degree in Figure 3.30 and to a greater degree in Figure 3.31 the tendon fascicles concentrate in two masses, a major dorsal tendon mass and a minor palmar one. In Figure 3.34 an intramuscular septum has emerged between these tendons. The transverse lamina has made contact with the fascial compartment and the dorsal tendon is led into a pericapsular position in the same manner as in dorsal II and IV. It is generally recognized in the literature that the palmar tendon will radiate into the transverse lamina and that only a minor portion is engaged in the formation of the wing proper. Another picture of dorsal I is found in Figures 3.95 and 3.97; here the palmar tendon is of fairly considerable size. More distal sections show that the thick dorsal tendon becomes entirely absorbed by the phalangeal base and, as usual, the outer anchor of the volar plate merges with the outer layers of this tendon complex.

General Discussion of Dorsal Interossei

The observations made so far seem to warrant the conclusion that a definite consistency exists in the internal arrangement of dorsal interossei IV, III and II and indeed no such conclusion could be reached without the support of these characteristic patterns seen within the muscles.

Dorsal IV and II, as already mentioned, are much alike, although we have the impression that the pattern common to both is more marked in dorsal IV where it presents its most elaborate, or most refined, expression. Basically, a dorsal interosseus is composed of a two-bellied dorsal portion and a palmar portion arising from the homonym metacarpal. It is important to note that tendon formation takes place in such a way that the two dorsal bellies converge upon tendon fascicles in the intramuscular cleft. Quite soon a main dorsal, an intermediate and a small palmar tendon can all be distinguished. The formation of the dorsal tendon proceeds in a whorl shape and mainly involves the radiodorsal quadrant. The palmar tendon obtains its fibres not only from the deep palmar muscle portion but also from the ulnodorsal belly. The incorporation of the interosseus into the metacarpophalangeal area is quite intriguing from a structural angle in the following ways: (1) the formation of an intramuscular septum as a marginal outer layer of the dorsal tendon; (2) the disappearance of the juxtametacarpal compartment wall in the dorsoradial quadrant, which places the dorsal tendon in juxtacapsular position; (3) the anchorage of the palmar tendon to the transverse intermetacarpal ligament through its own fibres and by means of a fibrous sling formed by the intermediate tendon; (4) the extension of the transverse lamina into the intramuscular septum; (5) the change of level of this lamina so that eventually a wing of the extensor assembly is formed.

Our conclusion is that both the insertion pattern of this muscle and its structural role in the constitution of the metacarpophalangeal region are closely related to the internal arrangement of the muscle. The same circumstances apply to dorsal II, although its structural refinement seems definitely less marked. Dorsal III is totally different internally from dorsal II and IV although, remarkably, its proximal base is identical with those of dorsal II and dorsal IV. Dorsal III resembles II and IV as far as the constitution of muscle bellies is concerned, where a two-bellied dorsal part and an additional palmar belly arise from the homonymous metacarpal, but no spiraling or whorling phenomena are seen in the dorsal tendon, this tendon eventually being represented by a bundle of rather discrete fascicles. A strong anchorage of various fascicles to the volar plate can be seen. No intramuscular septum is seen in this muscle, which is a remarkable observation because this septum shows a definite relationship to the spiraling of the dorsal tendon in dorsal II and IV.

As mentioned, no special analysis of dorsal I has been carried out since the structure of this muscle can be determined by micro-dissection and only a few sections were needed to confirm the massive phalangeal insertion of this muscle. A radiation of fibres into the transverse lamina was found in both series. Transverse series are not suitable for use in determining the number of fibres of the palmar muscle portion which pass into the wing of the assembly and so for this purpose we must rely on dissection.

General Summary of Dorsal Interossei

Dorsal interossei all have in common their dorsal bipennate origin, in addition to which they have a deep belly originating from the metacarpal of the ray to which they belong. It should be stressed that this deep belly does not behave entirely as a separate entity. In dorsal II and IV this belly forms part of the larger external muscle area lying outside the intramuscular septum; and it is this external area which includes a deep portion, which ultimately provides the wing tendons of these two muscles. Obviously the wing in the finger lies superficial to the phalangeal tubercle into which the dorsal bellies send their so-called phalangeal tendon. We have laid much emphasis on the internal structure of both these muscles which are so much alike and in particular on the formation of (1) the dorsal tendon in its whorl-like manner; (2) the intramuscular septum and (3) the wing tendon.

The incorporation of the phalangeal tendon into the pericapsular system and its relation to the external root of the volar plate also have been discussed. The radiations of tendons and their anchorage to the transverse intermetacarpal ligaments have been thoroughly studied and so has the shift of the transverse lamina which enables a wing to be formed. Delaminations from the wing system towards the phalangeal tendon are observed quite regularly.

In dorsal III, although the proximal picture of the muscle is basically the same, tendon formation progresses in a different manner. No whorling occurs in the dorsal tendon and there is no formation of an intramuscular septum so that later a multifasciculate wing is formed without a phalangeal insertion. In contrast, nearly the whole muscle of dorsal I contributes to the formation of a strong phalangeal tendon, only a palmar portion spirals round the phalangeal tendon mass and radiates into a transverse lamina; in this case the wing is almost entirely formed by the lumbrical.

3. THE DISTAL MIDHAND AREA

Conspicuous features of the midhand are (1) the gradual spreading of the flexor tendon layer; (2) the grouping together of the flexor profundus and the flexor sublimis for each finger; (3) the individualization of the lumbrical areas between the tendon areas and (4) the location of the nerves above the lumbricals. The latter process is followed by the formation of septa which join the palmar aponeurosis to the interosseous fascia. The palmar aponeurosis is a thick layer composed of longitudinal strands, locally superimposed on a fascial sheet which on the ulnar aspect becomes a strong transverse layer forming the ulnar compartment wall.

Figure 3.9 of *series no. 1899* is taken as the base of the proximo-distal analysis of the distal half of the palm, including the process of isolation of the fingers. At this level the interossei are seen to be fully developed and there is a most conspicuous tendon formation in the abductor digiti V, the opponens occupying only a limited area.

The deep ulnar nerve passes below the oblique head of the adductor pollicis. The abductor pollicis has become quite small and the opponens pollicis is near the distal end of its insertion. The flexor pollicis brevis is fully developed. The radial branch of the volar digital nerve of the thumb has just crossed the flexor pollicis longus tendon.

A glance at the palmar aponeurosis shows its extension into the skin of the thenar eminence and on the ulnar side its continuity as the ulnar wall of the flexor compartment can be seen. Notice that in a larger portion on the radial side the longitudinal fibre system is preponderant and only a few thin fascial strands lie below the impressive longitudinal tracts. In the ulnar portion related to the flexor tendons of the little finger, a transverse fibre system is most marked. The longitudinal system is represented here by only a few tracts. It seems beyond dispute that these longitudinal tracts also contribute to the ulnar wall of the compartment. In its turn this wall is continuous with the septum between the fourth palmar interosseus and the opponens digiti V. We will indicate the attachment of this ulnar compartment wall to the skin by means of a fibrous anchor, in the next chapter.

The flexor tendons for each finger are grouped together. The ulnar bursa entirely surrounds the deep fifth tendon. Along the superficial fifth tendon we observe a small cleft on its ulnar side. Both the superficial and the deep fourth tendon are each on the ulnar side and partially surrounded by a cleft. These clefts have just emerged. Clefts cannot be seen with certainty for the third and second fingers. The flexor pollicis longus tendon is surrounded by a cleft, except for a conspicuous mesotendineum. The peritendineal layers are embedded in loosely arranged connective tissue with the nerves, vessels and lumbrical muscles.

We will now follow closely the transformations that pertain to the palmar aponeurosis, viz. (1) its involvement in the process of the isolation of the fingers; (2) the formation of compartments in the palmar area, and (3) the formation of tendon sheaths.

It should be noted that at the level under consideration the palmar aponeurosis is anchored to the deepest corial layer; that these anchors compartmentalize the subcutaneous layer; that sweat glands are enclosed in these compartments, and further that at some places our observations allow us to speak of a subcorial layer.

The very earliest indication of a compartment, visible in Figure 3.10, lies around the tendons of the fifth finger and is the result of the formation of a septum between these tendons and the lumbrical muscle.

The layers of the aponeurosis have fused in this area and it is no longer possible to describe the septum between the tendons of the fifth finger and the adjacent lumbrical as being a continuity of either of the two layers of the aponeurosis. It is certainly not a formation derived exclusively from a transverse system.

Another septum starts to penetrate between the tendons of the third finger and the third lumbrical muscle. Locally, the fascial layers are strongly reinforced so that the palmar aponeurosis appears as a double layer at some places. This new septum is an extension of the deepest layer of the palmar aponeurosis. However, in sections proximal to this level it is by no means simple, if at all possible, to follow the superficial and the deep layers as individual entities. Further, the septum appears to contain transversely cut and hence longitudinal lying fibres.

The next septum to develop arises between the lumbrical of the middle finger and the long index tendons.

Thus we can see in this section partitions for (1) the long tendons of the little finger, (2) the long tendons of the ring finger flanked on both sides by a lumbrical, (3) the long tendons of the middle finger and their lumbrical, and (4) the long tendons of the index with their lumbrical. The development of the partition walls is accompanied by the more or less marked reappearance of the transverse layer of the palmar aponeurosis and by a concentration of the longitudinal fibres into strands which at this level are still somewhat irregular.

Examination of the origin of the partitions shows that the longitudinal system penetrating between the fibres of the transverse system contributes to their formation. We have already mentioned the longitudinal fibres present in a septum. We are now quite near to the metacarpophalangeal joint of the fifth finger and we can see that the intramuscular septum has considerably shortened and divided to allow the digital artery to pass behind the tendons of the fifth finger. The most ulnar of the palmar aponeurosis septa shows a distinct slope to the radial side, but this is not yet marked for the septum on the ulnar side of the tendons of the middle finger. Another partition wall now starts developing on the radial side of the index area. Here we observe a gradual closure of the flexor compartment around the radial volar nerve of the index and the ulnar pollex-nerve (Fig. 3.11). Soon, however, the pollex-nerve becomes enclosed in the thenar fascia. It should be noticed that the radial wall of the flexor compartment is not as dense a structure as the ulnar wall.

The distal palmar crease appears on the ulnar side of the fifth finger at the same time as the joint cavity of the little finger metacarpophalangeal joint appears. In a section such as Figure 3.11 we can clearly see components of the volar plate, the metacarpo-glenoidal ligament, extensions from the deep abductor tendons and extensions from both the transverse lamina and the abductor fascia.

As already mentioned, the distal crease is now crossing the fifth finger area. From the wealth of sweat glands in the area, the crease is seen to have been cut more or less tangentially over the flexor sheath of the fifth finger. The attachment of palmar aponeurosis fascicles in this skin area, hence around the crease, is a most conspicuous feature of this and adjacent sections.

Let us now see what happens in the other areas at the levels we are passing. A major point of focus is the appearance of two septa, one on each side of the tendons of the ring finger, then the synovial clefts are seen to have fused and now pass, as one, around both tendons. Special attention should be given to the relations within the compartment. The cleft has a wall, the peritendineum, a layer which is separated from the compartment wall by an areolar space. The picture in Figure 3.15 shows the septa as derivatives of the palmar aponeurosis, both layers of which seem to contribute to their formation, while a form of crossing takes place in the tendon area because the ulnar wall is formed by fibres from the radial side and the radial wall by fibres from the ulnar side. Again both septa are seen to contain longitudinal fibres. This same section shows the gradual reinforcement of the palmar interosseous fascia to what is recognized as the transverse intermetacarpal ligament. Let us now look closely at the situation in the fifth finger. The septum on the radial side of the flexor sheath of the fifth finger is inserted obliquely into the transverse intermetacarpal ligament and so forms a niche bordering on the synovial cleft in which vascular tissue is found.

We are now quite near the appearance of the tendon sheath of the little finger. A fibrous sickle, bordering immediately upon the synovial space, represents the true fibrous tendon sheath. *It is located within the compartment formed by the palmar aponeurosis. Some contribution from the compartment wall to the tendon sheath proper is certainly probable.* The sheath itself can be considered as a derivative of the volar plate (Fig. 3.12).

Where the crease moves over the fifth finger tendon sheath we find that the strong fibrofascial components of the envelope which are directly derived from the palmar aponeurosis have been stripped from the sheath. One should notice that a thin fascial layer persists around the tendon sheath and is separated from it by an areolar layer and *in this way the palmar aponeurosis does not cease to exist as a layer.*

While the tendon sheath moves gradually towards the midline of the fifth finger its formation can be followed step by step. The fibrous sickle we described above as the very beginning of a fibrous sheath and coinciding with the appearance of the joint cavity does not persist very long and it does not complete a half-circle. It is replaced by a new sickle which will surround the tendon entirely. The extension of this latter fibrous sickle progresses at the expense of the septum. These two structures are in contact at their tips and an exchange of fibres is certainly possible. This derived sheath, however, extends in close apposition to the peritendineal wall (Fig. 3.15).

The ulnar compartment wall has now been transformed into a thin fascial layer which is separated from the sheath proper by an areolar space. It is, however, important to pay attention to the radiations of the abductor fascial system into the subcutaneous space both proximal and distal to the distal crease. Analysis of the insertion of the abductor digiti quinti has shown the role of the transverse lamina in relation to the fascia between abductor and opponens and to the intramuscular laminae that direct the tendons into their periarticular position. A Figure such as 3.12 shows a most characteristic cross-section of this proximodistal process. In this section it can be seen that the distal crease, just appearing on the ulnar side, is firmly anchored to the dorsal superficial fascia, to the transverse lamina and to the abductor fascia. It is sometimes questioned whether true radiations of the abductor tendon are found in this anchoring system. However, somewhat distally, where the outermost tendons of the abductor are incorporated into the fascial system, it can clearly be seen that the anchoring system is to some extent part of this tendineal system, although it may not be a direct extension of the tendons. Figure 3.15 gives a good picture of the structural incorporation of the majority of the abductor tendons into a pericapsular system.

We have to return now to the point raised above, viz. the formation of the tendon sheath and its relation to fibrofascial envelopes. We will now follow the sickle-like tendon sheath that was seen in Figure 3.15. The dismantling of the compartment wall was well advanced on the ulnar side. At these levels, which are also levels of the distal crease and where the fibrous sheath starts appearing, the compartment loses its ulnar attachment to the volar plate; this means that its continuity becomes more marked with the fibrofascial layer in which the nerves are embedded and which belongs to the abductor tendon-fascia system (Fig. 3.13).

We recall here that on the radial side we saw a niche formed by the oblique insertion of the palmar aponeurosis septum. This niche is gradually replaced by the extension of the fibrous sickle into a rounded flexor tunnel. Basically, the fibrous tendon sheath develops *within* the *fascial* palmar aponeurosis compartment and to a certain extent the fibrous sheath replaces the sheath formed by the palmar aponeurosis. It is now relevant to observe what is happening to the palmar aponeurosis compartment, but this cannot be done without taking into account the extensions of the abductor compartment.

It is quite certain that the palmar aponeurosis fascicles which build up the compartment are firmly attached to the transverse intermeta-carpal ligament and also to the volar plate. Although continuities between the compartment wall and the fibrous sheath proper are seen, the individuality of the sheath is beyond doubt. It is well worth noting that the fibrous sheath first arises distal to the compartment, the latter being seen considerably proximal to the distal crease. By extending closely around the synovial cleft the fibrous sheath is gradually completed and the areolar space around it follows this fibrous formation. While the partition wall already mentioned becomes inserted into the transverse intermetacarpal ligament at an acute angle, the fibrous sheath is a structure rounded on both sides. There also takes place at this time a very strong development of the volar plate. At more proximal levels we saw the formation of the volar plate from the two metacarpo-glenoidal ligaments. At this level (Fig. 3.22) where the phalangeal base invades the metacarpophalangeal bundle, we see that the volar plate obtains an anchorage to the phalangeal base by means of both a deep and a superficial system. Both of these systems approach the phalangeal tubercle and together they encircle the tubercle from below. The superficial system is continuous with, or merges into, strata derived from the tendons of the abductor and from the intramuscular laminae which are, in their turn, derived from the transverse lamina.

It is also clear now that the more superficial abductor tendons, with their surrounding fasciae, radiate into the volar skin and that they encircle the ulnar vessels and nerve, so constituting the fascial envelope of the fibrous sheath. The completion of the fibrous sheath is clearly visible in Figure 3.22, where the distal crease lies over the lumbrical area adjoining the little finger. It may be observed in passing that the fourth palmar interosseus with its tendon is attached to the capsule of the joint. As the distal crease moves over the lumbrical area it absorbs the roof of this compartment, so that the lumbrical muscles, with the digital nerves and vessels, appear denuded in the area between the distal palmar crease and the basal digital crease, i.e. the webspace (Fig. 3.23).

One thing attracts our attention particularly: this is the relatively dense fibrous texture of the subcutaneous area over the fifth finger which is derived from the abductor area and also from a radial source, viz. the transverse intermetacarpal ligament below lumbrical IV. The closer we come to the phalangeal base, the thinner becomes the volar plate with the result that the flexor tendons glide on the palmar surface of the phalanx. The sheath in its turn again becomes very thin. In fact the two rounded sides of the sheath gradually cease to exist and the superficial layer of the sheath becomes the only fibrous covering. This means that niches are formed again, sharp niches in those places where proximally the rounded wall of the sheath previously had been located. These niches are rich in vessels. As the tendon envelope is interrupted at places, the vascular peritendineum which has reappeared is in fairly direct contact with subcutaneous layers (Figs. 3.27 and 3.28).

We are now close to the basal digital fold appearing on the ulnar side of the hand. While the fibrous sheath becomes thinner some strands of the most superficial covering gradually leave the tendon sheath layer and join the system of the subcutaneous fibrous tissue. This cannot take place, however, unless the areolar space around the tendon sheath becomes obliterated, which can be seen in Figure 3.26 while Figure 3.30 shows that there is an areolar space again formed around a tendon sheath which is seen to arise from the margin of the volar side of the phalanx. We are now faced with a second segment of the tendon sheath which will be termed the phalanx I segment. This segment is surrounded by a fascial layer derived from two sources, the compartment walls of the palmar aponeurosis and the metacarpophalangeal sheath.

As the basal digital fold crosses the fifth finger it takes attachment on both proximal and distal surfaces to the subcutaneous fibrous systems, which include the fibrous strands derived from the most superficial layers of the metacarpophalangeal sheath segment. After the strands have joined the subcutaneous layer, a new areolar space arises round that part of the tendon sheath which is derived from, or attached to, the phalanx. This delamination considerably reinforces the subcutaneous region, particularly the layer bordering the areolar space.

The fascial envelope of the tendon sheath is firmly anchored to the basal digital crease and is reinforced by contributions from the superficial member of the twin tendon of the fourth palmar interosseus (Fig. 3.30).

The digital nerves in the fourth intermetacarpal space are already somewhat separated from each other, and the common digital artery begins to divide. We see now a gradual reinforcement of a subcorial layer in the webspace which provides the natatory ligament.

Another inescapable phenomenon is the extension of fibrous skin anchors over the separating individual digital nerves, these being the first indication of the superficial lamina of the nerve-vessel sheath of the fingers.

Strong fibrous strands extend from the fascial envelope of the tendon sheath and pass into the subcorial fibrous system (Figs. 3.30 and 3.31). In Figure 3.31 and 3.33 fibrous strands are seen to extend from the subcorial layer towards a thin fascial layer that covers the diverging palmar nerve and artery on their palmar aspect. At this level there is some indication of a natatorial ligament emerging from the fascial hood around the sheath in the ring finger and passing ulnarwards. Doubtless the fibrous anchors just described originate in the same subcorial layer. As we come closer to the separation of the fingers these anchors move dorsally between the two finger areas and so establish contact with the fused layers of the nerve-vessel sheath. The fibres are observed to encircle a dorsal vein and then pass dorsally into the deepest layers of the subcutaneous fascia (Fig. 3.34).

The eventual separation of the fingers is prepared for by the emergence of dorsally placed arciform fibres which join the dorso-palmar systems described. These arciform fibres follow the developing dorsal indentation between the two fingers. The dorsal fold moves into a deeper position and only a slightly disordered mass of fibrous tissue remains between the two fingers. The interdigital fold is made up of dorsopalmar directed strands that are actually derivatives of the natatorial ligament on its palmar side and which radiate dorsally into the subcutaneous fascial system.

It seems advisable to look at what is happening with the tendon sheaths of the other fingers at more proximal levels. Naturally we can expect parallel phenomena. At the levels where the formation of septa is well on its way (Fig. 3.13) we also see the synovial clefts around the flexor tendons appearing. The formation of septa around the tendons of the fourth finger has already been mentioned. Transversely cut fibres in these septa indicate the presence of longitudinal fibres in them. The roof of the compartment shows a frank transverse course of fibres (Fig. 3.18) and close inspection reveals that these transverse fibres run towards the interosseous fascia in such a way that the longitudinal fibres are sandwiched between two layers of the transverse system. Gradually the transversely arranged system replaces the longitudinal fibres that obviously become inserted into the layer which can be termed the transverse intermetacarpal

ligament. A most conspicuous feature is the gradual reinforcement of
the compartment wall transforming it into a true fibrous sheath.
This process, however, is observed to occur only around the *ulnar*
aspect of the tendon where a rounded sickle-like sheath is formed
(Fig. 3.21) which is continuously reinforced *from* the *radial* side by
contributions from the transverse layer. On the radial side, however,
the compartment wall does not become rounded; a vascular niche is
formed instead, only possible because this compartment wall is
inserted into the deep fibrous layer at an acute angle. This process
takes place at levels of the metacarpal head (Fig. 3.23). The volar
plate is fully developed, the sheath segment formed so far is a part of
the volar plate and is attached to it by fibres surrounding the tendon
as well as by fibres joining this segment on the ulnar aspect (Fig.
3.25) from the transverse intermetacarpal ligament.

The distal crease is now crossing the sheath of the fourth finger
and the remainder of the longitudinal palmar aponeurosis strands is
absorbed by this crease (Fig. 3.25). One point calls for special
attention and this is the appearance of a fibrous subcorial layer in the
webspace between the fifth and fourth finger. This subcorial layer
presents as a proximal natatorial ligament. It is derived on the ulnar
side from the abductor tendon-fascial system and on the radial side it
seems that a strand from the palmar aponeurosis contributes to its
formation (Fig. 3.27).

At this point something happens that deserves close attention. The
fibrous sheath of the ring finger, that was certainly a continuity of
the palmar aponeurosis system, becomes disrupted and ceases to exist
and at the same time, a new fibrous spur emerges from the volar
plate (Fig. 3.30). This ulnar spur extends and replaces the fibrous
sheath of more proximal levels, gradually becoming sickle-shaped.
The original proximal sheath as such disappears and its fibrous
components are seen as an irregular layer around the new sickle-form,
separated from it by an areolar space. The surrounding fibrofascial
layer is inserted into the skin by fibrous anchors distal to the distal
crease. The sheath proper is rounded on all sides and is a structure
which belongs typically to the volar plate (Fig. 3.33). We could
expect that the fibrofascial envelope of the sheath distal to the
transverse intermetacarpal ligament should continue in a dorsal
direction, enclose the lumbrical and make contact with the transverse
lamina. It is certainly not surprising that radiations into the superficial fascial layers should exist. The distal crease lies now distinctly
radial to the lumbrical area between the fourth and third fingers.

A webspace extends on the palmar side of the nerves at some distance beyond the crease and the fibrous roof derived from the palmar
aponeurosis disappears over the nerves and vessels. The flexor
tendons of the third finger are still surrounded by a fibrous sleeve
derived from the palmar aponeurosis and it can be noted that there
is still an areolar space between the wall of the synovial cleft and the
sheath (Fig. 3.32). A fibrous sickle immediately bordering the synovial
cleft heralds the emergence of a true flexor tunnel derived from the
volar plate (Fig. 3.35) and while this is in progress, the webspace of
the third intermetacarpal space develops. The fully developed fibrous
sheath and webspace can be seen in Figure 3.36.

Before describing the ultimate division of the third webspace we must turn for a while to the transformations which are taking place in the tendon sheath of the ring finger. So far we have observed the metacarpophalangeal sheath section. The insertion of the volar plate that proceeds through the well-known anchoring systems encircling the basal tubercles of the phalanx, leads the ring finger tendon sheath to its distal end. A new section in close contact with the previous one arises from the lateral volar ridges of the first phalanx. It can be seen (Fig. 3.35) that fascial continuities arise from the end of the sheath of the ring finger in a layer that is separated from the phalanx I section of the sheath by an areolar space. Hence we can now see the classical picture of the longitudinal composition of a tendon sheath and the formation of fascial layers in the webspace area. The separation between the fingers is anticipated, as in the fourth interdigital space, by a dorsopalmar fibrous system that runs as a spur between the digital nerves and arteries of the adjacent sides of two fingers. This fibrous spur is derived from, or is part of, the fascial system around the tendon sheaths proper. It is worth noting again that we distinguish a metacarpophalangeal portion of a sheath derived from or forming part of the volar plate. This part of the sheath is surrounded by a fascial layer which is basically a continuity of the compartment of the palmar aponeurosis.

The formation of the sheath of the index can be followed in the same figures as that of the medius.

In both fingers the metacarpophalangeal joint is sectioned to show the full development of the volar plates. Figures 3.33 and 3.34 show for both fingers a sheath being derived from or, at least being in close relation with, the palmar aponeurosis. In both fingers this sheath is provided with a rounded ulnar wall and a radial niche.

At levels about Figure 3.35, again in both fingers, the sheath or sleeve derived from the compartment wall is replaced by a genuine metacarpophalangeal tunnel that presents primarily as a fibrous spur emerging from the volar plate. Again this sheath can be recognized by the fact that the synovial membrane is tightly attached to the inner side of the sheath and no areolar space intervenes between these two layers.

The sheath section in Figure 3.36 is complete for the medius and for the index. Figure 3.36 is also quite interesting in this respect as it shows here the first phalanx segment of the sheath in the ring finger, the metacarpophalangeal part in the medius and in the index fingers. The picture also shows the dorsal metacarpal veins.

DISCUSSION

An analysis of midhand cross-sections enables us to say that this area is characterized by a certain number of key-features.

The proximal base of the midhand is largely determined by the arrangement around the distal exit of the carpal canal. The transformation of the radial half of the carpal canal into the thenar musculature has been traced in some detail. The gradual substitution in a distal direction of the opponens pollicis by the fusing of the superficial flexor bellies and the spiraling of the deep flexor around the long flexor of the thumb represent the most conspicuous phenomena in this area. The hypothenar complex springs from the pisiform and from the ulnar wall of the carpal canal and this area also provides some features worthy of particular attention.

The phenomenon of the two layers of the opponens digiti V could be related to the course of the deep branch of the ulnar nerve. This branch passes between the two opponens layers and skirts the hamulus distally to gain the deep palmar space; this requires that the ulnar wall of the carpal canal be dissolved to allow the nerve to pass. Distal to this passage a new wall of the flexor compartment becomes established. At carpal, or basimetacarpal levels, palmar IV originates on the outer side of the distal exit of the carpal canal. Somewhat further on, an ulnar flexor compartment wall is formed on the outer side of this muscle. This also means that the muscle passes into the midpalmar space through the same opening as the nerve and artery. The deep branch of the artery passes into the midpalmar space by skirting the long flexor tendons, not by passing through the hypothenar eminence.

We have the impression that it is difficult anatomically to distinguish the flexor digiti V brevis, in contrast to the flexor pollicis brevis which presents a clear-cut anatomical entity. We wish to stress the difference between the complicated multitendinous abductor digiti V and the more simple abductor pollicis brevis. A distinction between dorsal and palmar interossei is perfectly reasonable, since all dorsal interossei are bipennate in their dorsal portion while some have a similarity of internal structure. Palmar interossei invariably take origin from one metacarpal only.

Dorsal II and IV resemble each other quite closely. We paid considerable attention to the formation of the dorsal tendon, its incorporation into the pericapsular strata, its final insertion into the phalangeal base and its relation to the external root of the tendon sheath. The division of the muscle by an intramuscular septum and the location of this septum fitted logically into the structural and spatial arrangement of the muscle. The transverse lamina is formed by the merging of this intramuscular septum with the palmar extension of the intertendinous fascia.

We also laid emphasis on the formation of the wing tendon, especially on its anchorage to the transverse intermetacarpal ligament and to the way it fuses with the transverse lamina to form a wing proper.

The third dorsal, as we have said already, behaves like a dorsal interosseus as far as its proximal base is concerned. It turns out, however, that the conspicuous tendon formation of dorsal II and IV does not take place in quite the same way in dorsal III which would seem to preclude a division of the muscle as found in II and IV; and indeed dorsal III formed a multifasciculate wing tendon. Dorsal I occupies a more or less separate place among the dorsal interossei. Each palmar interosseus arises from one metacarpal only but they display differences among each other. The second muscle seems to be the most complicated for its inner structure has some resemblance to a dorsal interosseus; it is seen to present two tendons in our material so far and in one of our two specimens the tendons behaved as a dorsal III, which means that they took part in the formation of one multifasciculate wing tendon. In the other specimen the dorsal tendon became a phalangeal tendon and the palmar one a wing tendon. Palmar IV, though fairly complicated in its inner structure, differs from palmar II. In one series we found the formation of a twin tendon, one of the tendons becoming inserted into the phalanx, the other one becoming a wing tendon. In the second series we could only trace a wing tendon, though there were conspicuous extensions into the volar plate. Palmar III is definitely the simplest of them all: we found only a wing tendon and no extensions into the volar plate.

The arrangement in the midhand is largely determined by the grouping of flexor tendons alternating with the lumbrical muscles and with the digital nerve and vessels.

The alignment of digital structures in the ray of the finger is also reflected in the structural arrangement of the palmar aponeurosis. The spreading of the palmar aponeurosis with its ulnar and radial extensions must be mentioned. The radial extension into the subcorial layers of the thenar eminence shows up in marked contrast to its anchorage to the ulnar side of the ulnar flexor compartment wall; this point will be discussed in more detail in Chapter 4. It can also be seen that the palmar aponeurosis develops proximally as a multilayered structure containing extensions from the palmaris longus as well as from the flexor retinaculum.

In Chapter 4 we will comment in more detail on the role of the tongue-like ligament derived from the pisohamate bundle in the formation of the palmar aponeurosis. Formation of septa, concentration of the superficial longitudinal layer into languettes, emergence of true tendon sheaths at metacarpophalangeal level and relationships between tendon sheaths and palmar aponeurosis compartments all deserve close attention. The webspaces and the structural and spatial implication of the separation of the digits from the midhand have been given due consideration.

We hold the view that both longitudinal and transverse fibres share in the formation of the septa. It should be remembered that the septa begin proximally with a free border sloping towards the interosseous fascia. Cross-sections reveal longitudinal fibres in the septa, particularly where the septa appear as projections on the deep aspect of the palmar aponeurosis. There seems to be no doubt that the transverse system contributes to the septa in the region between the transverse creases of the palm. This relationship is decided unequivocally in cross-sections and by dissection. We have already noted particularly in the proximal area that the palmar aponeurosis appears as a duo- or multilayered structure, and the finding will be given due attention in a microdissection of the midhand.

We are faced with the problem of the transition of the palmar aponeurosis compartments into tendon sheaths proper at the distal crease, as we approach the webspaces. We believe that it is sensible to reserve the term 'tendon sheath' for those fibrous structures which border the cleft around the tendon, without the interposition of an areolar space between the synovial membrane and the fibrous layer. For this reason we prefer to speak of 'compartments' in those circumstances where such an areolar space does exist. This happens to be the situation at levels between the transverse creases of the palm, where synovial clefts exist which are surrounded by compartment walls derived from the palmar aponeurosis, and areolar spaces are interposed.

Adjacent to the compartment the sheath that surrounds the tendon from metacarpophalangeal levels onwards comprises a number of segments. We are inclined to distinguish the following segments in a tendon sheath:

(a) the metacarpophalangeal segment;
(b) the phalanx I segment;
(c) the proximal interphalangeal segment;
(d) the phalanx II-distal interphalangeal segment.

It is obvious that in this chapter only segments (a) and (b) have been described.

The most proximal segment of the tendon sheath proper, the metacarpophalangeal segment, is strictly a derivative of the volar plate, which in its turn forms part of the ligamentous system of the joint. It is striking to find that this segment extends around the cleft and lies in close contact with the synovial membrane. It is certainly probable that continuities exist between the compartment derived from the palmar aponeurosis and the flexor tendon tunnel proper. On the other hand a free proximal border of the tunnel is not at all exceptional and this will be referred to again in the microdissections and in the horizontal and sagittal series.

It is obvious that the distal continuity of the palmar aponeurosis presents as a major problem in this area of transition. Generally speaking, the languettes have a tendency to anchor themselves to the subcorial system just beyond the distal crease. It is not surprising, of course, that every now and then we see distal extensions of this system. Another point to be made is that the compartment is still present as a fascial layer distal to the emergence of the flexor tunnel where it surrounds the sheath proper and is separated from it by an areolar layer. This so-formed fascial hood is quite thin locally and actually represents the layer of the palmar aponeurosis. It is not surprising therefore that this layer should contain longitudinal strands derived from the longitudinal palmar aponeurosis layer and that these strands, like the longitudinal components of the septa, pass towards the transverse intermetacarpal ligament where they are inserted in the niches between lumbricals and tendon sheaths. It is quite understandable that fibres of the compartment wall, especially around and just beyond the distal crease, may extend towards the skin, instead of rounding the compartment wall.

The presence of a fascial hood around the sheath seems to be the basic picture at metacarpophalangeal level. At the same time the webspaces open up because the transverse system does not occur beyond the distal palmar crease. The nerves and artery have no covering layer except for the fatty pad of the space, until, towards the base of the phalanx, the arrangement changes. A basic feature is the anchorage to the phalangeal base of the volar plate, including the tendon sheath. The volar plate embraces each of the two basal tubercles of the phalanx with an external and an internal fibrous root, each acting as an anchor. The external root blends proximally with the pericapsular layers and with the phalangeal interosseous tendon layer when this exists. Through this anchorage not only does the volar plate establish a connection with the first phalanx, but the tendon sheath becomes suspended from the phalangeal base. This state of the metacarpophalangeal tendon sheath suggests that the next tendon sheath segment should be looked upon separately, because it is not suspended from the phalanx but fuses into its lateropalmar ridges. This segment might be termed the phalanx I segment. It is not so surprising that this transition is accompanied by a continuation of the metacarpophalangeal sheath layer as a fascial layer around the phalanx I segment, though this does not always occur to the same degree. Remembering that the former sheath segment was surrounded by a fascial layer, it seems logical that the two should fuse.

The natatorial ligament is a reinforcement in the subcorial system and anticipates the separation between the fingers. This system is in contact with the fascial hood around the phalanx I tendon sheath which often becomes reinforced again at these levels. Furthermore we see extensions from the natatorial ligament on the inner side of the nerves and arteries of a webspace. In this way nerve-vessel sheaths are formed, one for each side of a finger. We might say that a fibrous spur from the natatorial ligament extends dorsally between the digital nerves and arteries. This fibrous spur blends dorsally with fibrous layers formed from the subcutaneous fascia and local delaminations of the transverse laminae. The ultimate division between neighbouring fingers is preceded by arciform fibres which support the dorsal interdigital fold.

We note here that little attention has so far been paid to the extension of fibrous strands from the metacarpophalangeal region into the finger; the strands contribute to the digital band. This point will be described in later chapters.

SUMMARY

In a summary of the transformations taking place between the carpus and the bases of the fingers the following features are relevant:

(a) The grouping of tendons for each finger and the interposition of the lumbrical muscles, the artery and nerve;

(b) the formation of palmar aponeurosis septa with participation of both longitudinal and transverse components;

(c) the transformation in the thenar, hypothenar and interossei columns;

(d) the emergence of flexor tunnels, basically within the layer of the palmar aponeurosis compartment or its fascial extension;

(e) the more or less continuous transition of the metacarpophalangeal sheath segment into the segment of phalanx I;

(f) the role of the natatorial system in the division of the fingers and its relation to the fascial hood around the tendon sheath of phalanx I.

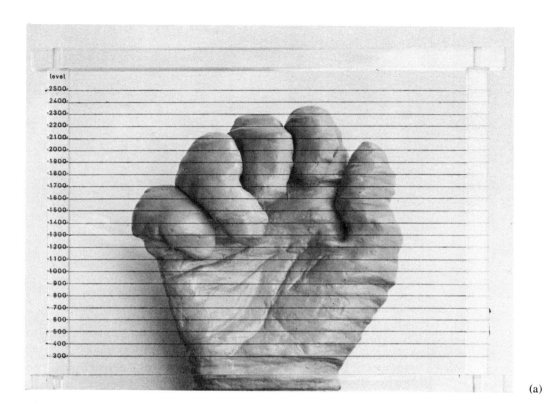

(a)

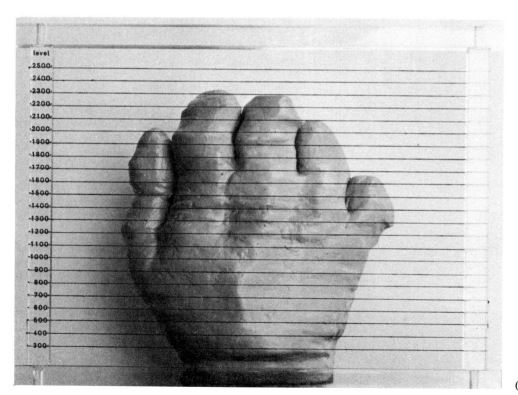

(b)

Fig. 3.0 (negs. 25689 and 25690) Reconstruction of the hand of *series no. 1899*. These pictures will help to locate sections by means of numbered levels.

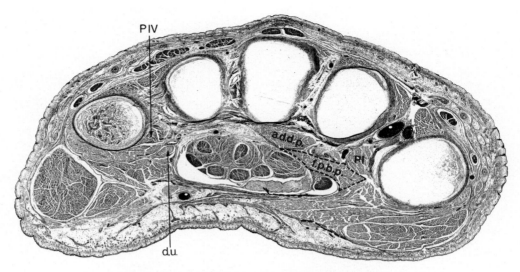

Fig. 3.1 (*Series no. 1899*; neg. 22506). Level: 739. Section at basimetacarpal level. Attention should be given to various layers in the palmar area, the flexor retinaculum, the palmaris brevis tendon and the deep and superficial layers of the palmar aponeurosis. The deep ulnar nerve is at the edge of the ulnar wall of the tunnel. The thenar area is composed of the abductor, the opponens, the proximal tips of the superficial flexor (indicated by dotted lines), the adductor, the deep flexor and palmar interosseus I; P I = palmaris I; P IV = palmaris IV; add.p. = adductor pollicis; f.p.b.p. = flexor pollicis brevis profundus; d.u. = deep branch of the ulnar nerve.

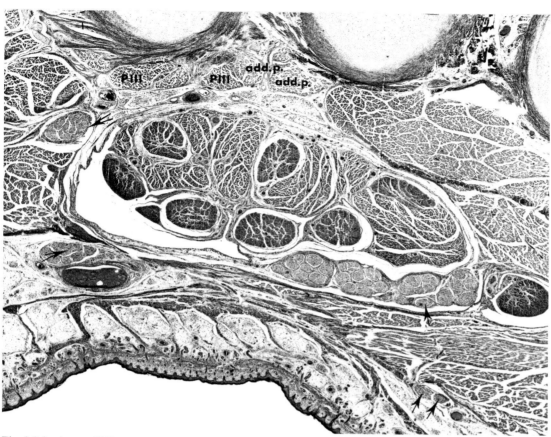

Fig. 3.2 (*series no. 1899*; neg. 13324). Level: 774. The carpal tunnel at the distal border of the flexor retinaculum. The ulnar bursa still shows considerable extension. All superficial tendons remain surrounded by synovial clefts. Note the thin wall of the cleft around the fifth finger. The areas of origin of palmar III and the adductor are indicated. Arrows: the recurrent branches of the median nerve. Double stemmed arrows: the superficial and deep branches of the ulnar nerve. P III = palmaris III; add.p = adductor pollicis.

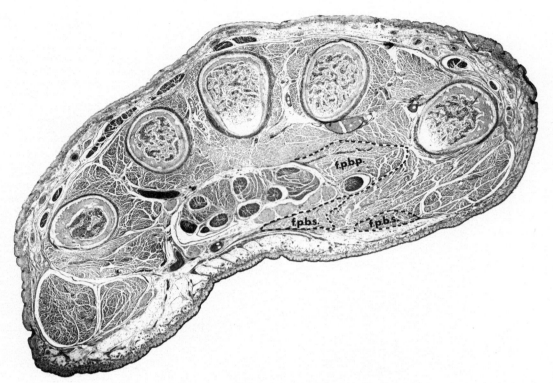

Fig. 3.3 (*series no. 1899*; neg. 13316). Level: 830. Section through the distal border of the flexor retinaculum. After the deep ulnar nerve passes over palmar IV, a new septum arises between this muscle and the opponens digiti V. In the thenar area muscular areas have become apparent which originated from the dotted lines indicated in Fig. 3.1. They represent the superficial part of the flexor pollicis brevis. The ulnar bursa gradually withdraws from between the superficial (IV and V) and the deep tendons (IV and V and the lumbrical). The synovial spaces around the superficial tendons narrow. f.p.b.p.= flexor pollicis brevis profundus; f.p.b.s.=flexor pollicis brevis superficialis.

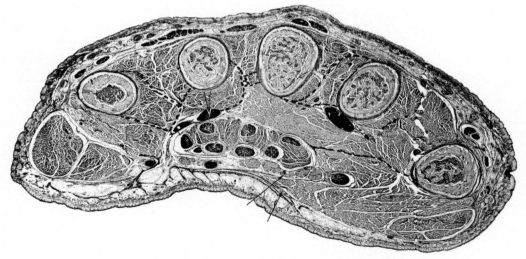

Fig. 3.4 (*series no. 1899*; neg. 18852). Level: 869. Section at proximal midhand level. Further retraction of the ulnar bursa. The superficial tendons are now only partially surrounded by a cleft. The radial artery crosses the second metacarpal. The double-stemmed arrow represents the perforating artery of Fig. 3.3. The other two arrows indicate the recurrent branch of the median nerve.

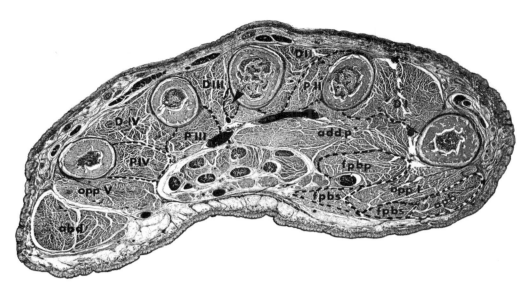

Fig. 3.5 (*series no. 1899*; neg. 18853). Level: 913. Section at proximal metacarpal level. Reclosure of the flexor compartment on the ulnar side. The synovial clefts around the second and third sublimis tendons have disappeared. A grouping of the tendons to each finger is quite conspicuous now. The arcus profundus passes the third metacarpal. Distal to this passage additional adductor bundles originate from the second and third metacarpals. Arrow: the additional area of dorsal II. abd. = abductor digiti V; opp.V = opponens V; P IV = palmaris IV; D IV = dorsalis IV; P III = palmaris III; D III = dorsalis III; P II = palmaris II; D II = dorsalis II; D I = dorsalis I; add.p = adductor pollicis; f.p.b.p. = flexor pollicis brevis profundus; f.p.b.s. = flexor pollicis brevis superficialis; opp.I = opponens pollicis; a.p.b. = abductor pollicis brevis.

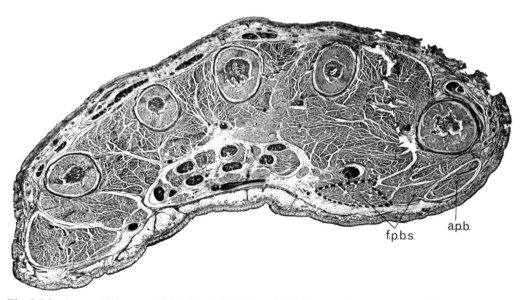

Fig. 3.6 (*series no. 1899*; neg. 18854). Level: 973. Synovial clefts are only present around each of the tendons of the fifth finger. A local bursa has developed between the deep tendon of the ring finger and the fourth lumbrical. The two hypothenar areas distal to the opponens have merged into one, the abductor area. Tendon formation in this area is well on its way. The deep flexor of the pollex starts to spiral around the long flexor tendon to join the superficial flexor. f.p.b.p. = flexor pollicis brevis profundus; a.p.b. = abductor pollicis brevis.

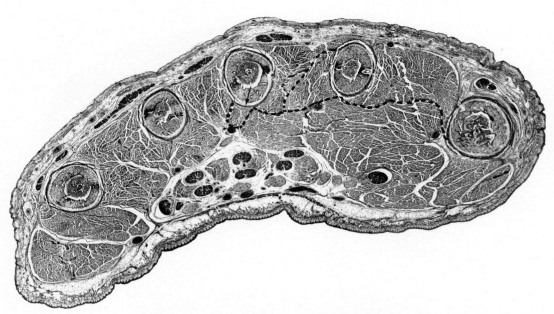

Fig. 3.7 (*series no. 1899*; neg. 22508). Level: 999. Section at proximal metacarpal level. The satellite area of dorsal II (arrow) will soon pass below the adductor with the deep branch of the ulnar nerve.

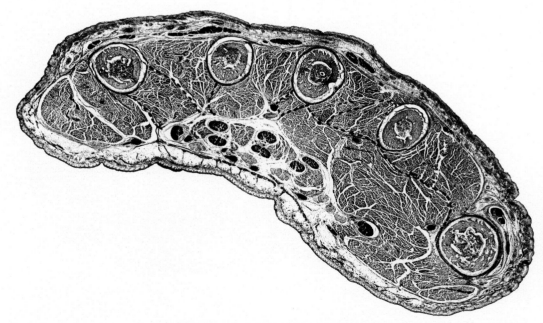

Fig. 3.8 (*series no. 1899*; neg. 18855). Level: 1015. Section at proximal metacarpal level. The grouping of the tendons with the lumbrical of each finger is now quite evident. The twisting of the deep flexor pollicis brevis around the long flexor pollicis is a marked feature. The local bursa between the deep tendon of the ring finger and the lumbrical extends also along the superficial tendon. Adjacent to this there seems to be the beginning of a cleft around the superficial tendons of the index and the fourth fingers. The adductor no longer originates from the second metacarpal. Flexor bundles have slipped below the abductor pollicis brevis. Note the course of an ulnar branch over the adductor area towards the deep flexor (arrow).

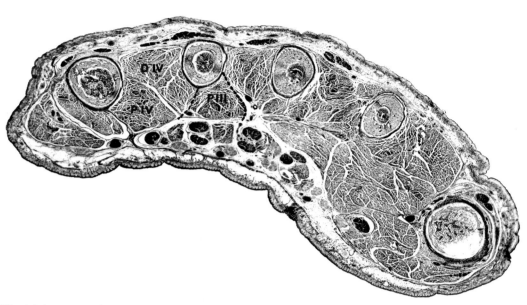

Fig. 3.9 (*series no. 1899*; neg. 21644). Level: 1078. Section at midmetacarpal level. The palmaris brevis has just disappeared from the cross-section. The spiral course of the deep flexor pollicis posterior to the long tendon is nearly completed. The radial digital nerve of the pollex has just crossed the long tendon. The opponens pollicis is near the end of its insertion and the abductor of the thumb will soon be incorporated into the extensor assembly of the thumb. The flexor pollicis touches the radial wing deep to the abductor pollicis. The adductor no longer originates from the third metacarpal. The deep ulnar nerve passes the free border of this muscle. The palmar aponeurosis radiates into the skin of the thenar. Tendon formation in the abductor area of the hypothenar is a conspicuous feature. Tendon formation starts in the area of interosseus IV. Next to the bursa lying between lumbrical IV and the ring finger tendons there seem to be new clefts developing close to each of the tendons of this finger. The anchorage of the ulnar flexor compartment wall is well seen. The palmar aponeurosis radiates into the skin of the thenar area. The radial nerve of the thumb just crosses the tendon. P IV = palmaris IV; D IV = dorsalis IV; P III = palmaris III.

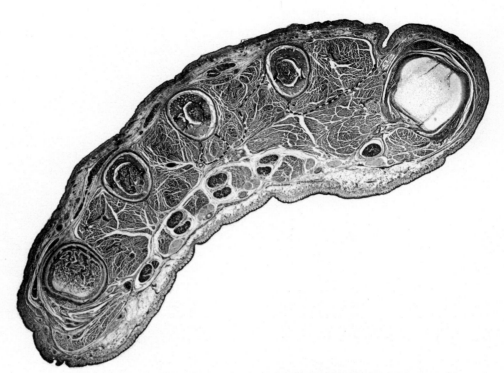

Fig. 3.10 (*series no. 1899*; neg. 13321). Level: 1156. Section at midmetacarpal level. A partition wall, derived from the palmar aponeurosis, has penetrated between the long tendons of the fifth finger and the fourth lumbrical. The common digital artery is incorporated into the intermuscular septum of the fifth metacarpal. The opponens digiti V is almost entirely inserted into the fifth metacarpal. The tendons of the abductor digiti V are in juxtacapsular position. Note the wing of the assembly on both ulnar and radial sides of the thumb and the convergence of flexor bundles in the base of the capsule. In dorsal IV, tendon formation is apparent in the dorsal area.

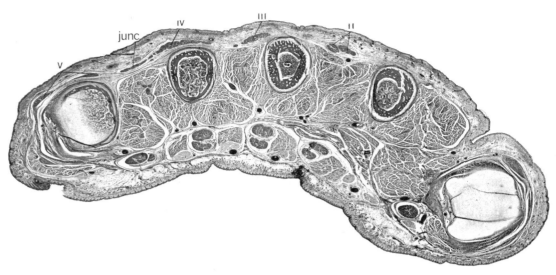

Fig. 3.11 (*series no. 1899*; neg. 21643). Level: 1191. Section at midmetacarpal level. The metacarpophalangeal joint of the little finger is cut. The distal palmar crease has made its appearance on the ulnar side. Note the lateral and basal origins from the metacarpal head of the ligaments composing the palmar pad. The fifth finger tendons are almost entirely surrounded by the ulnar bursa. The ring finger tendons are partially surrounded by a cleft. The deep, long tendon of the middle finger has a synovial cleft around it and so does the superficial index tendon. A septum is now present between lumbrical III and the long tendons of the finger. The interossei areas are indicated by dotted lines. Roman numerals indicate the related tendons. junc.=junctura tendineum.

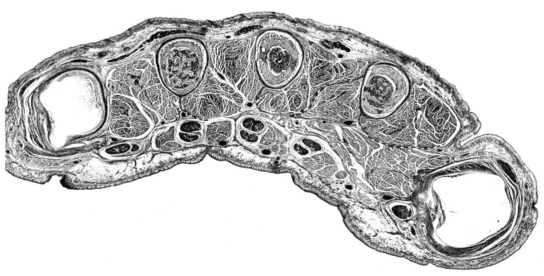

Fig. 3.12 (*series no. 1899*; neg. 21642). Level: 1213. The anchorage of the distal palmar crease by extensions from the abductor compartment in the fifth finger. Note the emergence of a fibrous sickle from the volar plate which lies in direct apposition to the synovial cleft. In various interossei, tendon formation is well advanced. The flexor pollicis brevis and the adductor pollicis concentrate at their respective sites of insertion. Note the further development of synovial spaces around the flexor tendons.

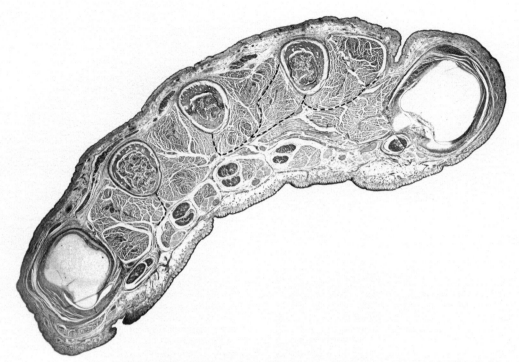

Fig. 3.13 (*series no. 1899*; neg. 13319). Level: 1229. Section at midmetacarpal level. As a result of the emergence of an areolar layer around what will become the tendon sheath, the palmar aponeurosis layer does not continue into the volar plate of the little finger (cf. previous figures): it keeps its continuity into the abductor fascia. Sesamoid bones have appeared in the capsule of the metacarpophalangeal joint of the thumb. Observe the extension of the adductor, while the flexor brevis has been entirely absorbed by the sesamoid bone. Tendon formation is marked in dorsal IV.

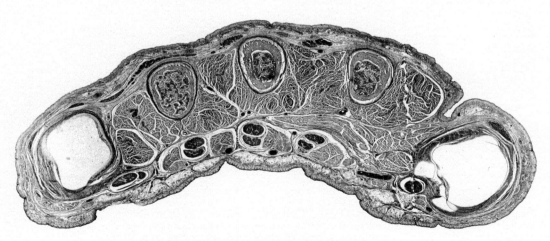

Fig. 3.14 (*series no. 1899*; neg. 24001). Level: 1243. Cross-section through the midhand. The metacarpophalangeal joints of both thumb and fifth finger are cut. Formation of septa from the palmar aponeurosis is well on its way.

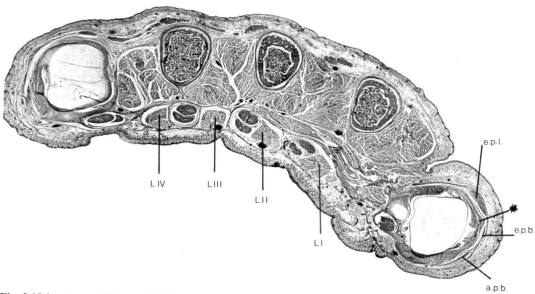

Fig. 3.15 (*series no. 1899*; neg. 21640). Level: 1278. Section at distal metacarpal level. The distal palmar crease lies just over the tendon sheath of the fifth finger. In dorsal IV, tendon formation is quite conspicuous in the dorsal area. L IV=lumbricalis IV; L III= lumbricalis III; L II=lumbricalis II; L I=lumbricalis I; e.p.l.=extensor pollicis longus; e.p.b.=extensor pollicis brevis; a.p.b.=abductor pollicis brevis; * for explanation see text.

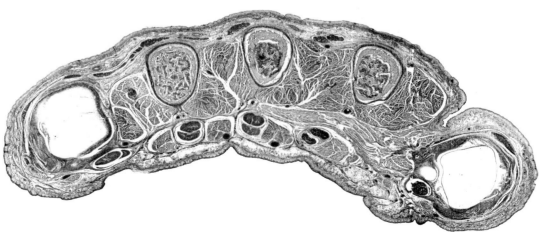

Fig. 3.16 (*series no. 1899*; neg. 24002). Level: 1280. Cross-section through the metacarpophalangeal joint of the thumb and the little finger. Tendon formation in various interosseous areas is clearly visible (cf. Fig. 3.17).

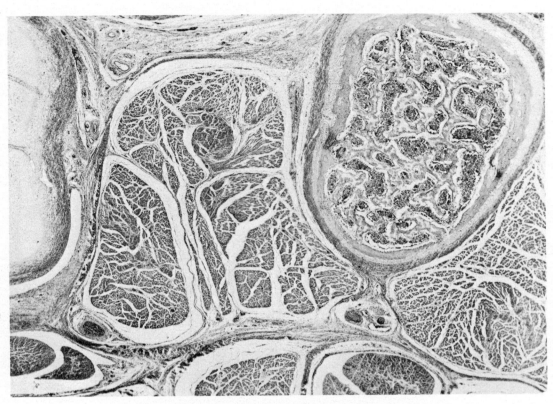

Fig. 3.17 (*series no. 1899*; neg. 14075). Level: 1281. A cross-section of the fourth intermetacarpal space. A fine example of whorling in the tendon of dorsal IV. Note the fascicles of the dorso-radial quadrant which do not take part in the dorsal tendon. In palmar IV both a major dorsal tendon and clustered palmar fascicles are visible. Finally in palmar III an H-like tendon formation can be seen.

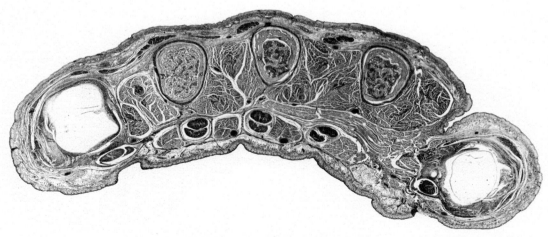

Fig. 3.18 (*series no. 1899*; neg. 24003). Level: 1294. Cross-section through the midhand. The distal palmar crease has just passed the fifth ray. The abductor pollicis brevis and extensor brevis are leaving the wing layer of the extensor longus.

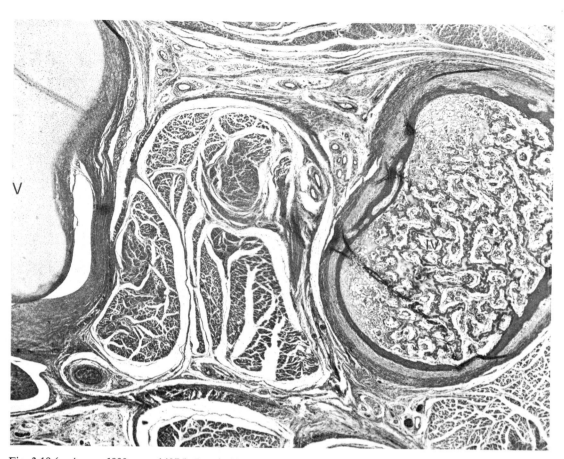

Fig. 3.19 (*series no. 1899*; neg. 14076). Level: 1316. The fourth intermetacarpal space.
In dorsal IV the intramuscular septum continues into the juxtametacarpal fascial wall.
Note the fascicles of the dorso-radial quadrant. In palmar IV the dorsal tendon becomes
attached to the juxtametacarpal compartment wall. V=fifth metacarpal; IV=fourth
metacarpal.

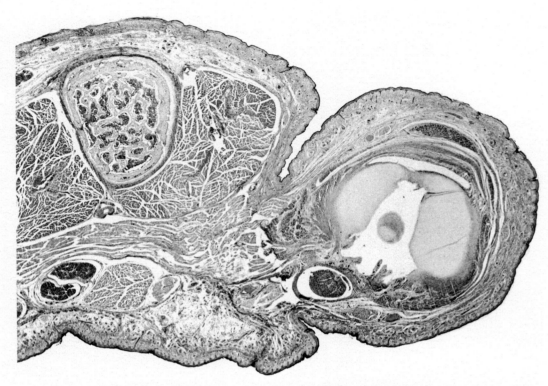

Fig. 3.20 (*series no. 1899*; neg. 23999). Level: 1323. Section through the phalangeal base of the thumb. Note the relative positions of the extensor pollicis longus and the extensor pollicis brevis. Tendon formation starts in dorsal interosseus I.

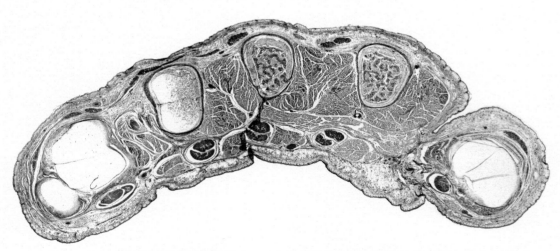

Fig. 3.21 (*series no. 1899*; neg. 22502). Level: 1336. Cross-section through the phalangeal base of the thumb. Conspicuous tendon formation in various interossei areas (cf. Fig. 3.22). Note the extension of the areas of dorsal II and III. In dorsal IV the dorsal tendon is now in a juxtacapsular position. In the thumb bundles from the abductor and the extensor brevis have left the wing and will soon be inserted into the base of the phalanx. The ulnar wing remains rather well-developed. The adductor again contacts the third metacarpal.

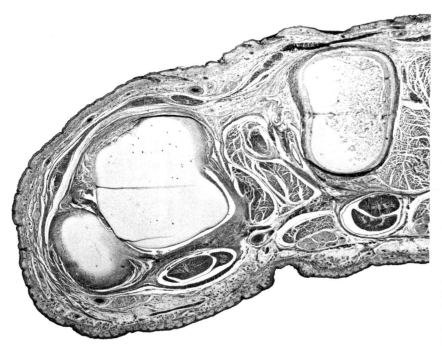

Fig. 3.22 (*series no. 1899*; neg. 13331).
Level: 1336. Cross-section of the fourth
intermetacarpal space. The disappearance
of the juxtacapsular compartment wall in
palmar IV has caused the main dorsal
tendon of this muscle to become
structurally related to the ligaments and
volar plate.

In dorsal IV the dorsal tendon is in a
juxtacapsular position. In the little finger
the tendon sheath, derived from the
volar plate, completely encircles the
tendons. An areolar space around this
sheath separates it from the fascial
envelope in which we found radiations
from the abductor insertion area. The
distal palmar crease has reached
the fourth lumbrical. Observe also the
attachment of the volar plate to the
phalangeal tubercle.

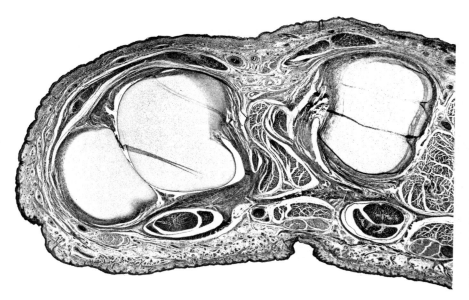

Fig. 3.23 (*series no. 1899*; neg. 13333).
Level: 1363. The distal palmar crease now
lies well over the fourth lumbrical and
takes up its roof, so that the lumbrical
emerges in the webspace. In palmar IV
two tendons run on both sides of a fibrous
anchor derived from the main dorsal
tendon.

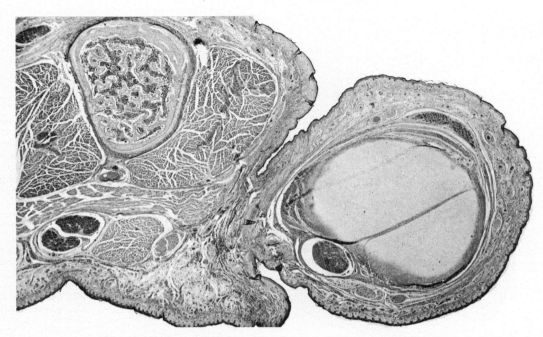

Fig. 3.24 (*series no. 1899*; neg. 24000). Level: 1363. Proximal section through the first phalanx of the thumb. The extensor brevis rejoins the longus layer.

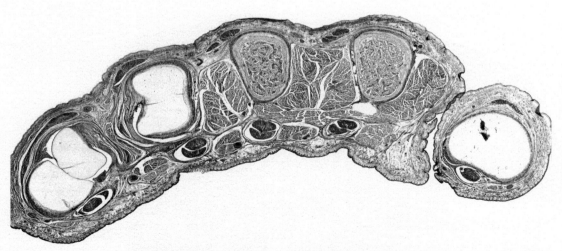

Fig. 3.25 (*series no. 1899*; neg. 22503). Level: 1401. The thumb is just isolated from the midhand. Interossei areas are clearly defined. A dorsal and a palmar tendon are visible in palmar II. See Fig. 3.26 for palmar IV and dorsal IV.

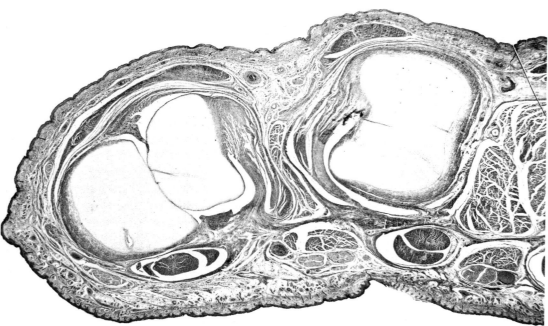

Fig. 3.26 (*series no. 1899*; neg. 13335). Level: 1401. In dorsal IV the main dorsal tendon is incorporated in juxtacapsular strata. The palmar tendon is situated on the outer side of the transverse lamina. In palmar IV the deep, dorsal tendon is suspended from the metacarpal head by pericapsular layers, while the palmar tendon forms part of an infratendineal fascial system.

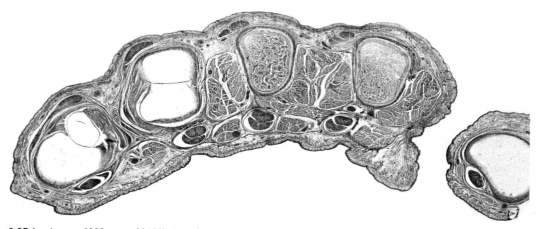

Fig. 3.27 (*series no. 1899*; neg. 22510). Level: 1425. Tendon formation in various interossei is well under way. The deep component of the twin tendon of palmar IV is suspended from the metacarpal head, its superficial partner appearing continuous with infratendineal layers. In dorsal IV the palmar extension of the palmar, superficial tendon should be noted. In palmar II tendon formation is specific in both dorsal and palmar portions. For further details of the fourth interspace see Fig. 3.28.

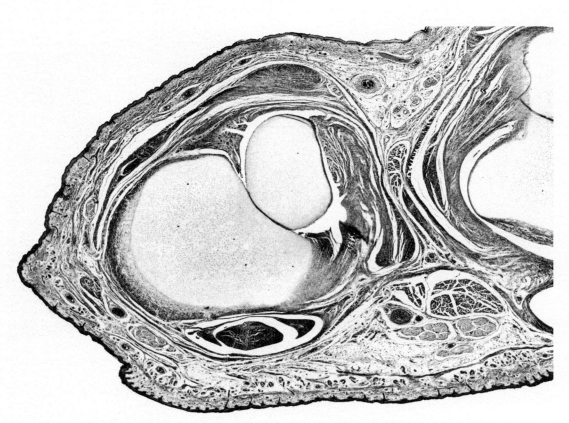

Fig. 3.28 (*series no. 1899*; neg. 13337). Level: 1425. Section through the fourth intermetacarpal space. On the ulnar side the rounded sheath of the fifth finger has disappeared and a vascular niche has taken its place. A delaminated superficial layer of the flexor sheath becomes part of the fascial envelope and encircles the artery and nerve on the ulnar side of the finger. The basal finger fold is already visible on the ulnar side. Note the natatorial-like reinforcement of the subcorial layer. In dorsal IV the deep tendon lies as a twin structure on the inner side of the transverse lamina. In palmar IV the deep tendon is still suspended from capsular layers.

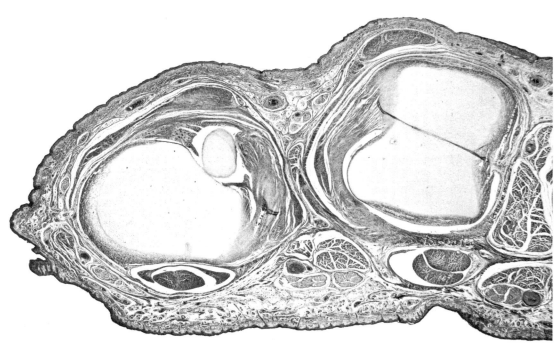

Fig. 3.29 (*series no. 1899*; neg. 13338). Level: 1438. In the fifth finger the ligament layer and the deep component of the twin tendon of palmar IV become invaded by the phalangeal base. The superficial tendon forms a wing here. In dorsal IV all components of the palmar tendon complex are inserted into the transverse intermetacarpal ligament.

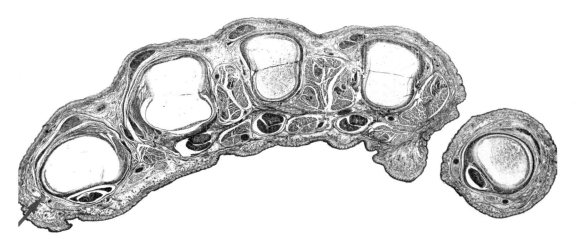

Fig. 3.30 (*series no. 1899*; neg. 22512). Level: 1473. In palmar IV the deep tendon has become inserted into the phalangeal base, while the superficial one is forming the wing of the assembly. In dorsal IV the phalangeal tendon is juxtaposed to the ligaments while the superficial tendon presents as the free border of the ulnar wing. Furthermore we see in palmar III a tendon in the palmar niche, in dorsal III a dorsal tendon, in dorsal II a thick dorsal tendon and a minor palmar one, in palmar II a major palmar tendon and a minor dorsal one and, lastly, in dorsal I we can see a dorsal elongated tendon cluster. At this level the basal digital crease begins passing over the little finger. The anchorage of this crease to the fascial system is most conspicuous. Observe the longitudinal bundle in relation to both this fascial system and to the wing of the little finger assembly (arrow).

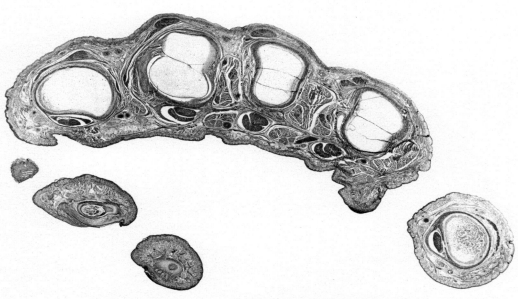

Fig. 3.31 (*series no. 1899*; neg. 24004). Level: 1497. Section through the distal midhand area. The basal digital crease passes over the little finger. The palmar roof of the webspace is formed by the reinforced subcorial system, the natatorial ligament. In dorsal IV part of the wing tendon delaminates to join the phalangeal tendon complex. In palmar III we see a tendon in the ulno-palmar niche of this compartment. Two tendons are visible in palmar II. A dorsal and palmar tendon complex can be distinguished in dorsal I.

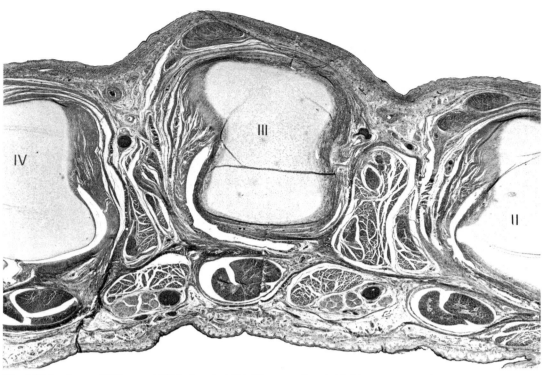

Fig. 3.32 (*series no. 1899*; neg. 16012). Level: 1546. The second and third intermetacarpal spaces. In palmar II the dorsal tendon is in closer apposition to the capsule. The major palmar tendon remains outside the transverse lamina. In dorsal II the major dorsal tendon becomes surrounded by a layer which will become an intramuscular septum. Tendon formation in the palmar area takes place in the palmar juxtametacarpal niche. In dorsal III all the dorsal tendons are anchored to the volar plate. In palmar III a tendon is visible in the palmar juxtametacarpal niche. Roman numerals indicate the corresponding metacarpals.

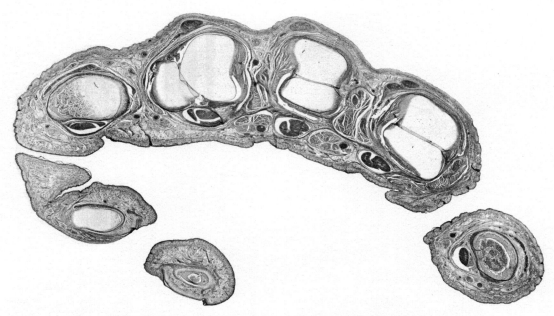

Fig. 3.33 (*series no. 1899*; neg. 24007). Level: 1549. Transverse section through a distal midhand level. Notice the strong fibrous junctions between the subcorial natatorial ligament and the fascial covering of the nerves and vessels. For tendon formations in various interosseous areas see Fig. 3.32.

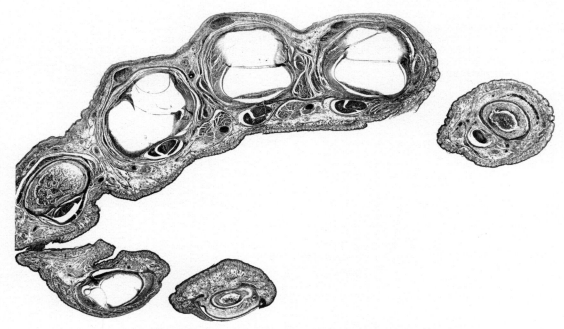

Fig. 3.34 (*series no. 1899*; neg. 22513). Level: 1594. Section close to the distal end of the fourth interdigital space. Dorso-palmar fibres can be seen in this area. The wing of the little finger has incorporated a portion of lumbrical IV. The interosseus palmaris on the radial side of the ring finger is a fairly simple club-like tendon, here it is in apposition to the transverse lamina. The radiations into the volar plate of the tendon complex of dorsal III, including the transverse lamina, are quite marked. Dorsal II shows the typical division into a dorsal phalangeal tendon and a volar wing tendon complex. Palmar II has already lost its dorsal tendon into the juxtacapsular layers. The palmar tendon lies in close apposition to the transverse lamina. Dorsal I shows one fairly massive dorsal tendon and a minor palmar one.

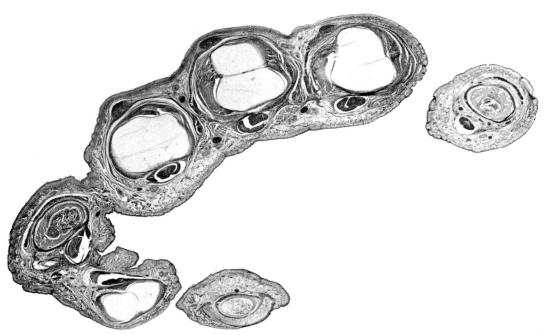

Fig. 3.35 (*series no. 1899*; neg. 16015). Level: 1646. Cross-section through the webspaces and through the first phalanx of the thumb. The palmar tendon of palmar II has become rounded off from the transverse intermetacarpal ligament. The tendon fascicles of palmar III have become incorporated into the wing. In dorsal III the wing tendon is nearly completed. In dorsal II the phalangeal tendon draws closer to capsular layers. In dorsal I the two tendons are separated from each other by the transverse lamina.

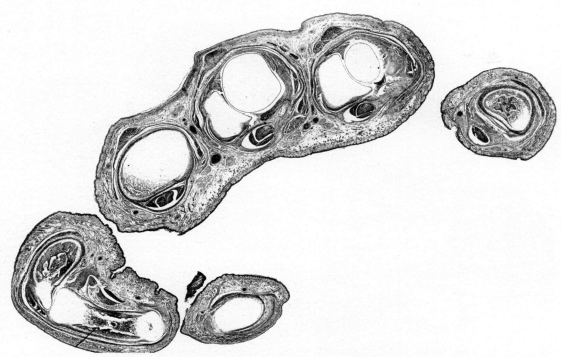

Fig. 3.36 (*series no. 1899*; neg. 22514). Level: 1730. The two wings of the extensor expansion of the ring finger are now rounded at their volar tips. The fascial system around the osteofibrous sheath of phalanx I of this finger holds the nerve-vessel bundle and is in intimate contact with the subcorial system in the basal digital crease. The ulnar wing of the middle finger expansion has incorporated all the fascicles of dorsal III; a portion of lumbrical III has some structural relation to the dorsal tubercle of the phalangeal base. On the radial side the phalangeal tendon of dorsal II is juxtacapsular in position. The wing tendon portions, including lumbrical II, still run lateral to the transverse lamina. The ulnar wing of the index has incorporated the palmar tendon of palmar II. On the radial side the major part of interosseus I is juxtacapsular in position. The wing will soon shift to the lumbrical.

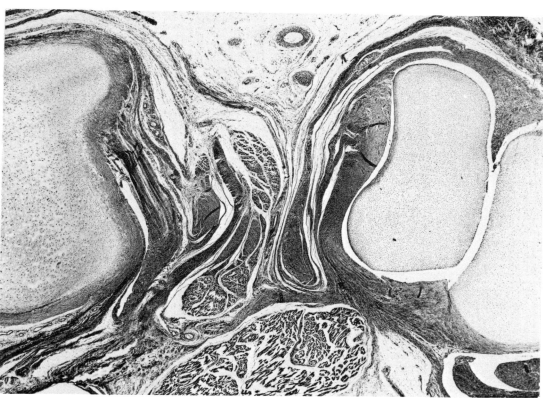

Fig. 3.67 (*series no. 1452*; neg. 13716). Level: 798. Enlargement of the fourth intermetacarpal space of Fig. 3.66. The joint cavity of the metacarpophalangeal joint of the ring finger is now in the cross-section. The main part of the transverse lamina continues into the lateral wall of the compartment (cf. Fig. 3.69). The formation of pericapsular layers derived from the dorsal tendon is clearly visible. In the volar ulnodorsal area the elongated intermediate tendon, a main volar tendon and the fascicles of the volar area of Fig. 3.64 are visible which all now collect upon the main volar tendon or skirt its lateral side. The tendon of palmar IV exfoliates fibres to its surroundings.

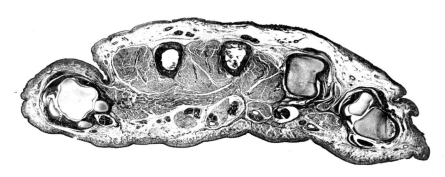

Fig. 3.68 (*series no. 1452*; neg. 12899). Level: 811. Section through the midhand. The base of the phalangeal base of the thumb has appeared in the section. Both sesamoid bones are visible. The wing belonging to the extensor longus is a fibrous sheet which blends with the capsule volarly and is also continuous with subcorial layers. Notice the strong fibrous systems of the capsule to which the whole extensor brevis and flexor brevis system belong. A rounded knob on the ulnar wing becomes conspicuous. Tendon formation in dorsal III concerns the main dorsal area. In this area we might distinguish a dorsal tendon cluster and a palmar tail.

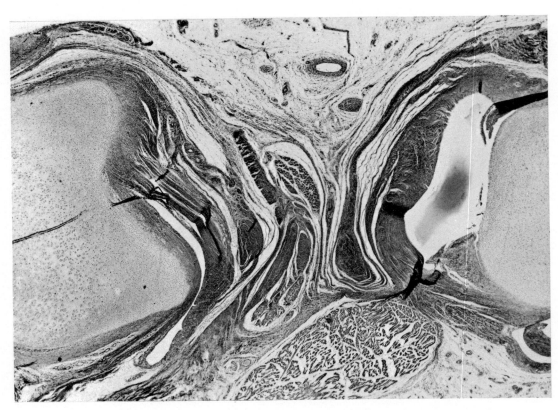

Fig. 3.69 (*series no. 1452*; neg. 13726). Level: 820. Section through the fourth intermetacarpal space. In dorsal IV the transverse lamina and intramuscular septum tend to become one stratum. The dorsal tendon is now a deep juxtacapsular tendon. Notice the continuity of the infratendinous fascia in pericapsular layers derived from the muscle. The intermediate tendon has elongated and extends into the transverse intermetacarpal ligament. For palmar IV see Fig. 3.67.

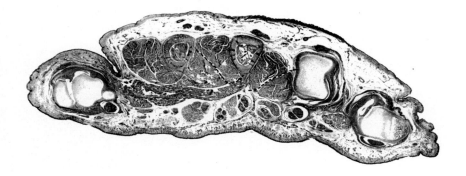

Fig. 3.70 (*series no. 1452*; neg. 12898). Level: 828. Cross-section about half way in the midhand. In the thumb the phalangeal base invades the capsular system. See Fig. 3.71 for the situation in the fourth intermetacarpal space.

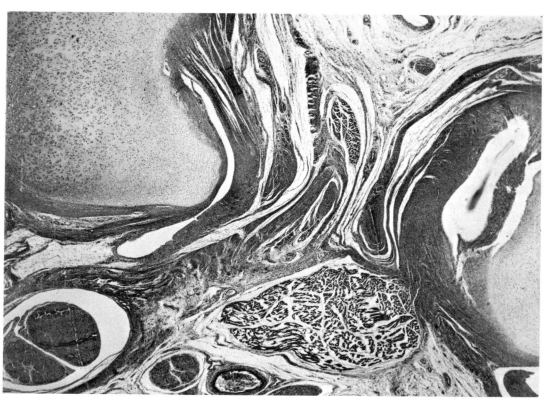

Fig. 3.71 (*series no. 1452*; neg. 13261). Level: 828. Section of the fourth intermetacarpal space. Dorsal IV and palmar IV are close to their insertion. Through elongation of the intermediate tendon and of the fascicle lateral to the main palmar tendon a complete sling is formed around the latter. In palmar IV we see exfoliation of the wing tendon into pericapsular layers.

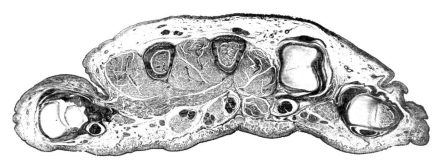

Fig. 3.72 (*series no. 1452*; neg. 12901). Level: 846. Section at a distal metacarpal level. In this picture the extensor longus wing is seen to be separate from the base of the phalanx. The ulnar wing is still fairly strong. In dorsal IV the transverse lamina has moved into line with the inner loop of the sling of the superficial tendon. In dorsal III we see clearly a major dorsal tendon and a palmar tail. A sagittally placed tendon cluster is apparent in palmar II. Note the origin of the adductor pollicis from the third metacarpal.

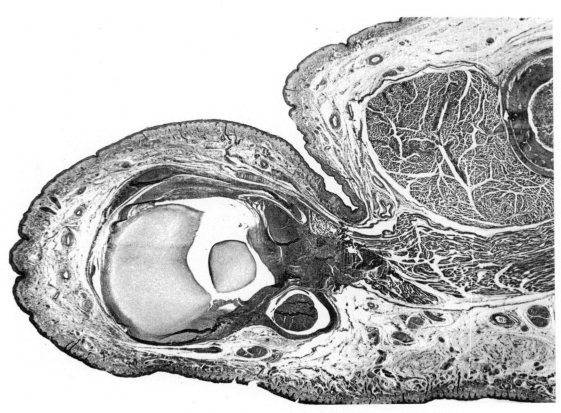

Fig. 3.73 (*series no. 1452*; neg. 23998). Level: 853. Section through the metacarpophalangeal joint of the thumb. Thick tendon masses run along the distal continuity of the ulnar sesamoid. The ulnar wing is still provided with a palmar knob.

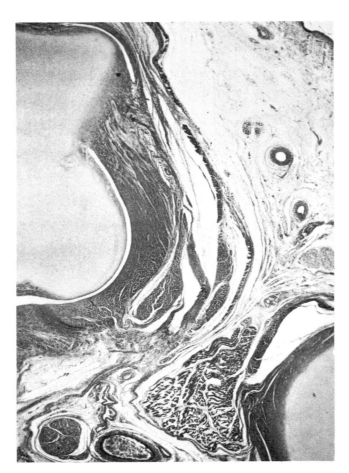

Fig. 3.74 (*series no. 1452*; neg. 13260). Level: 891. Detail of the situation on the ulnar side of the ring finger. The inner loop of the sling of the palmar tendon has become free from the transverse lamina and joins the pericapsular system in which we see the phalangeal tendon core. The wing tendon is a twin structure composed of the palmar tendon core and the top of the sling. The transverse lamina gives strong fibres which pass lateral to this system towards the volar side. Lumbrical IV is in the process of forming the radial wing of the extensor assembly.

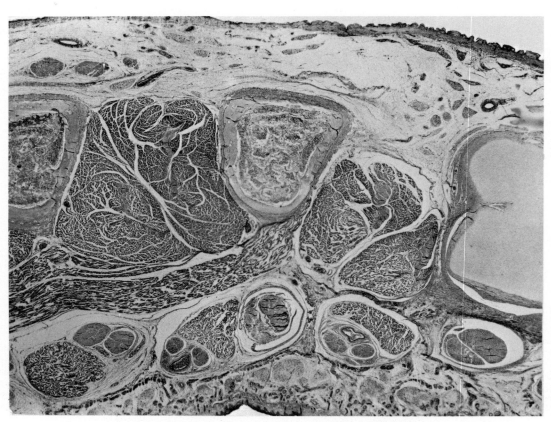

Fig. 3.75 (*series no. 1452*; neg. 14995). Level: 893. Interossei around the medius and palmar III. In dorsal III tendon formation in the main two-bellied area has led to dorsal and palmar tendons, the latter being also a rounded structure. The additional radial palmar area is still free of tendons.

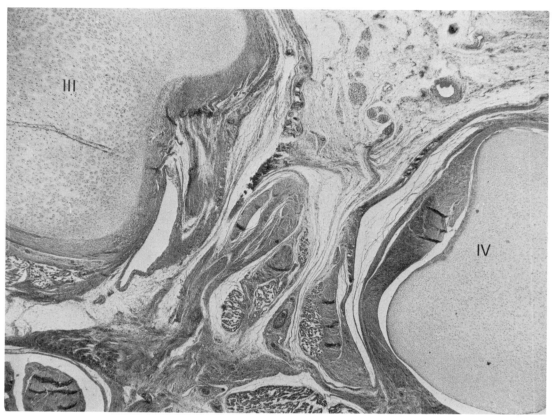

Fig. 3.82 (*series no. 1452*; neg. 15000). Level: 1013. The third intermetacarpal space. Formation of the wing is nearly completed in palmar III. The main dorsal tendon of dorsal III is anchored to the volar plate (cf. Fig. 3.79). III = metacarpal III; IV = metacarpal IV.

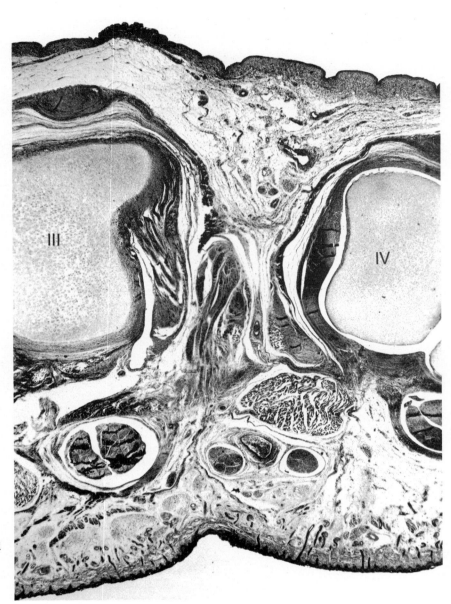

Fig. 3.83 (*series no. 1452*; neg. 16640).
Level: 1027. The third intermetacarpal
space. Anchorage to the volar plate of the
fascicles of the main dorsal III tendon.
The juxtametacarpal fascicles have replaced
the transverse lamina. The tendon of
palmar III has now moved into the
stratum of the transverse lamina. III=
metacarpal III; IV=metacarpal IV.

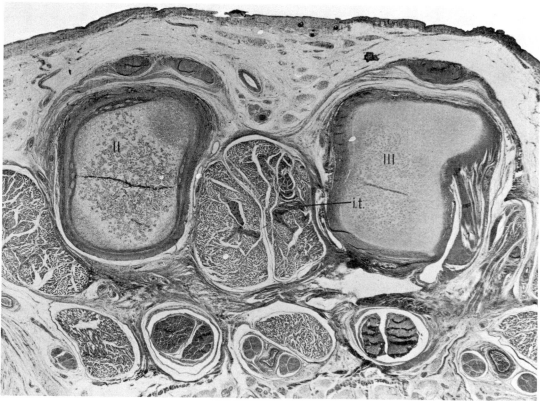

Fig. 3.84 (*series no. 1452*; neg. 14999). Level: 1032. The second and part of the third intermetacarpal spaces. The palmar tendon complex of dorsal III has also become anchored to the transverse intermetacarpal ligament. In dorsal II a marked dorsal tendon, an intramuscular layer as well as intermediate (i.t.) and palmar tendons are all visible. The major dorsal tendon in palmar II is easily seen, with the flat palmar tendon perpendicular to it.

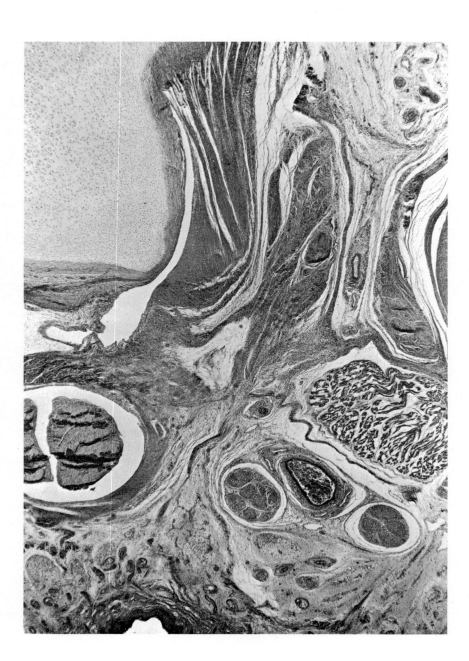

Fig. 3.85 (*series no. 1452*; neg. 15028).
Level: 1045. The third intermetacarpal
space. One of the palmar tendons of
dorsal III is anchored to the transverse
intermetacarpal ligament.

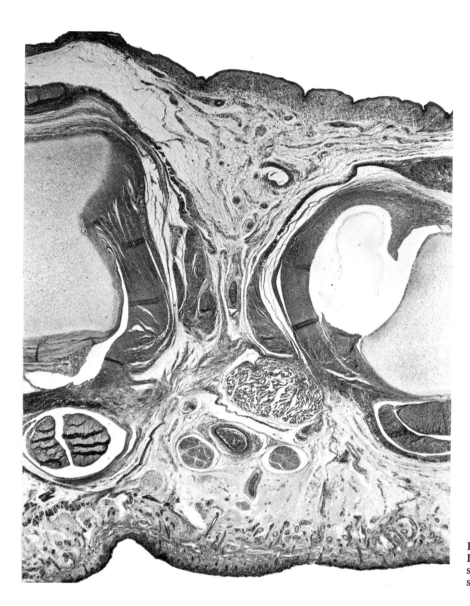

Fig. 3.86 (*series no. 1452*; neg. 16641).
Level: 1057. The third intermetacarpal
space. All tendons of dorsal III are now
suspended from the transverse lamina.

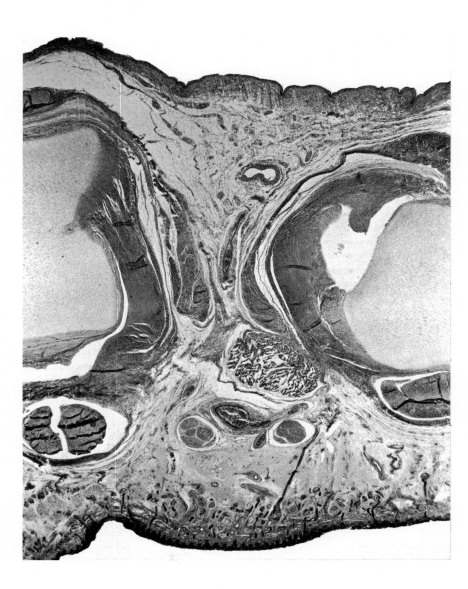

Fig. 3.87 (*series no. 1452*; neg. 16642).
Level: 1068. Section through the third
intermetacarpal space. The fascicles of
dorsal III expand into the wing.

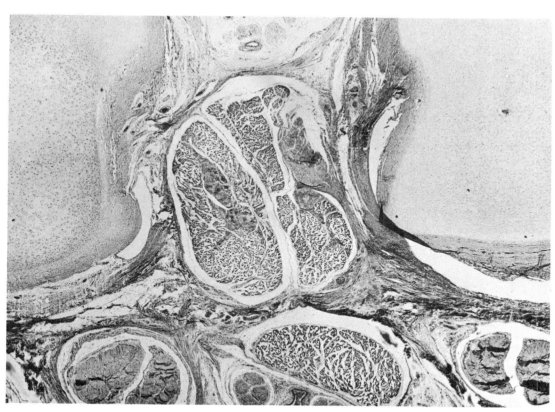

Fig. 3.88 (*series no. 1452*; neg. 23726). Level: 1074. The interossei of the second intermetacarpal space. Two tendons are visible in palmar II, a dorsal and a palmar. Dorsal II shows the typical picture of a dorsal tendon in the dorso-juxtametacarpal quadrant, an intramuscular septum blending with the compartment wall and a muscle area occupying the remaining three quadrants. The intermediate tendon of Fig. 3.84 and the intramuscular septum have merged into one layer which continues palmarwards in the juxtametacarpal compartment wall.

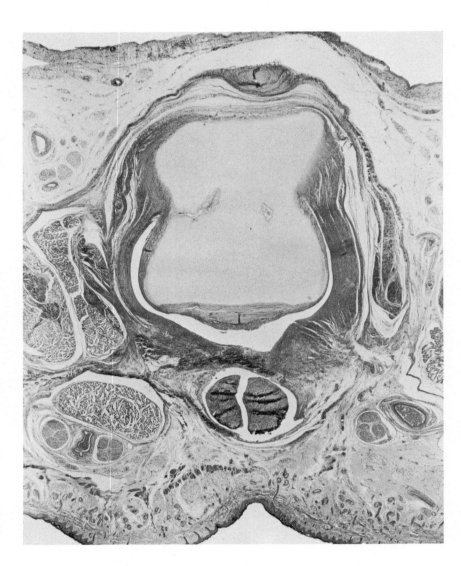

Fig. 3.89 (*series no. 1452*; neg. 15029).
Level: 1085. The two dorsal interossei of
the third ray and palmar II. In the latter
two major tendon masses can be
distinguished. In dorsal II the dorsal
tendon comes into a juxtacapsular
position. Note the intramuscular septum
and the conspicuous palmar tendon. In
dorsal III all tendons are suspended from
the transverse lamina.

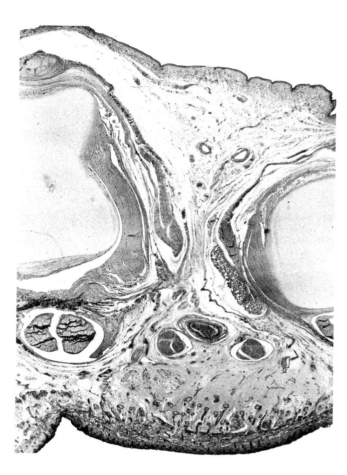

Fig. 3.90 (*series no. 1452*; neg. 16643).
Level: 1102. Section through the third
intermetacarpal space. In dorsal III
tendon fascicles fan out to form the wing.
In palmar III the lumbrical joins the wing.

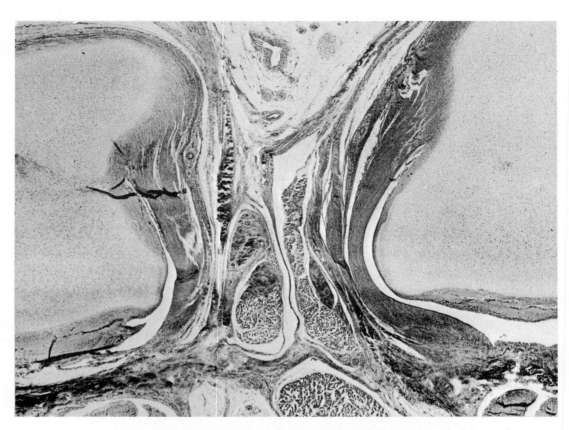

Fig. 3.91 (*series no. 1452*; neg. 23727). Level: 1127. Section through the second intermetacarpal space. In dorsal II we see a pericapsular tendon and another running on the outer side of the transverse lamina. In palmar II an intramuscular septum has developed, which merges with the juxtametacarpal compartment wall in a palmar direction.

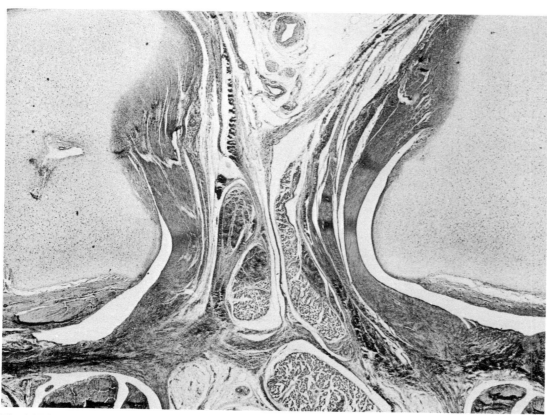

Fig. 3.92 (*series no. 1452*; neg. 23991). Level: 1140. The second intermetacarpal space. The juxtametacarpal compartment wall in the dorsal half becomes conspicuously thin in palmar II. In dorsal II the picture is typical of a phalangeal tendon in a pericapsular position and a palmar wing tendon.

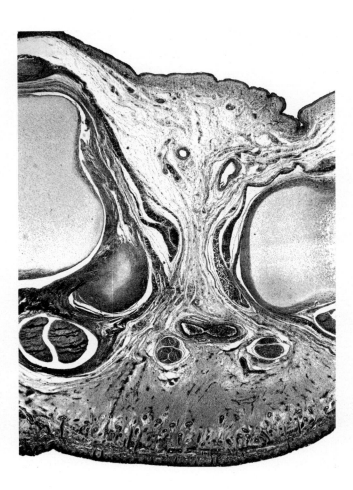

Fig. 3.93 (*series no. 1452*; neg. 16644).
Level: 1143. Section through the third
intermetacarpal space. In the wing on the
ulnar side of the medius the
multifasciculate appearance of dorsal III
can still be recognized.

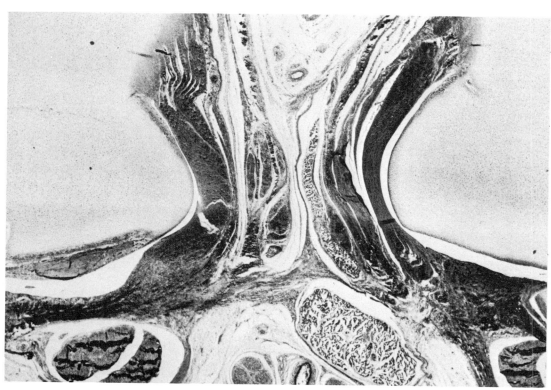

Fig. 3.94 (*series no. 1452*; neg. 23993). Level: 1170. Section through the second intermetacarpal space. In dorsal II fascial structures join the superficial or palmar tendon to the palmar ligaments. In palmar II the juxtacapsular compartment wall has vanished.

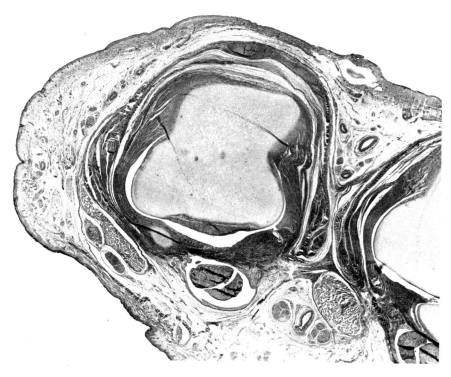

Fig. 3.95 (*series no. 1452*; neg. 24246). Level: 1181. Section through metacarpal II and the second intermetacarpal space. Notice the two parts of the tendon complex of dorsal I, a deep and a superficial tendon. In palmar II a multifasciculate tendon forms the wing. A deep pericapsular tendon and a superficial one separated by the transverse lamina can be distinguished in dorsal II.

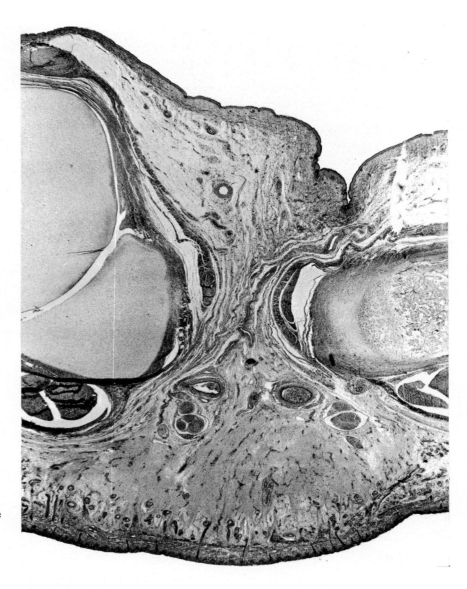

Fig. 3.96 (*series no. 1452*; neg. 16645).
Level: 1186. Section through the webspace
between III and IV. Note the anchorage
of the metacarpophalangeal sheath
around the basal tubercle of the phalanx
of the medius.

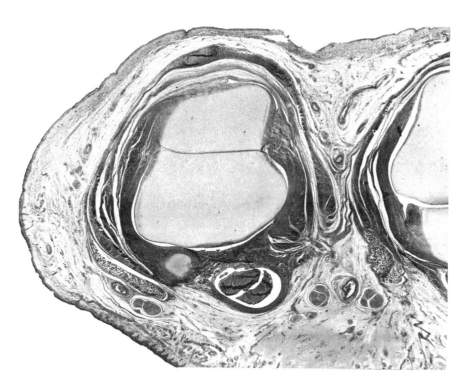

Fig. 3.97 (*series no. 1452*; neg. 24247).
Level: 1221. Section through metacarpal II
and through the second intermetacarpal
space. The tendon fascicles of palmar II
become increasingly concentrated into one
wing. In dorsal II the tendons are
continuous with extensions of the tendon
sheath. In dorsal I the superficial and deep
tendons can be clearly seen.

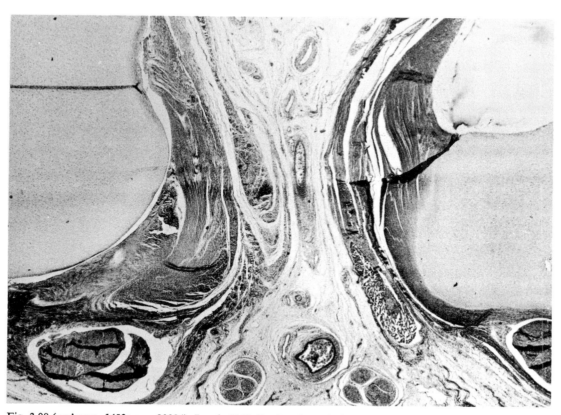

Fig. 3.98 (*series no. 1452*; neg. 23994). Level: 1254. Section through the second
intermetacarpal space. The base of the phalanx of the middle finger has been sectioned.
In dorsal II the layer of the phalangeal tendon has become continuous with the outer
anchor of the tendon sheath.

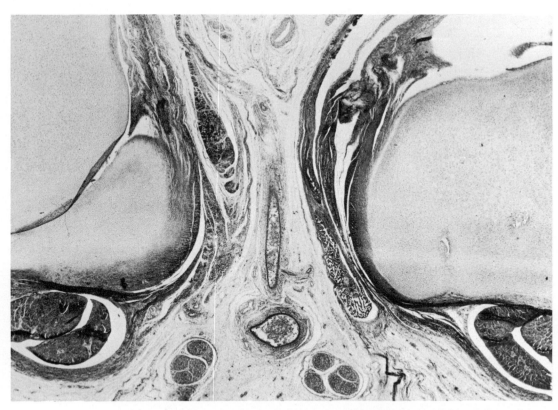

Fig. 3.99 (*series no. 1452*; neg. 23995). Level: 1269. The base of the first phalanx of the medius is seen invading the phalangeal tendon of dorsal II and the outer anchor of the tendon sheath.

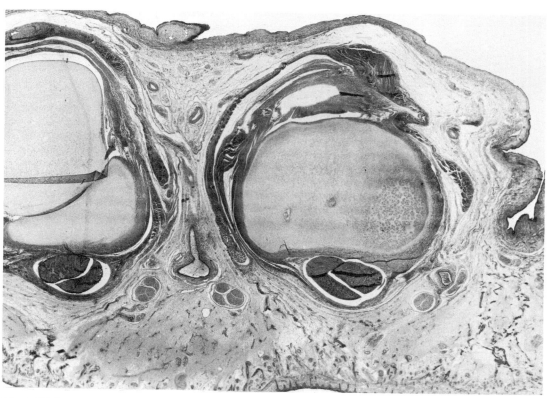

Fig. 3.100 (*series no. 1452*; neg. 24248). Level: 1277. Section through the second intermetacarpal space. The anchoring system of the tendon sheath of the index is separate from the wing tendon. In dorsal II the phalangeal tendon and the tendon sheath system merge into each other.

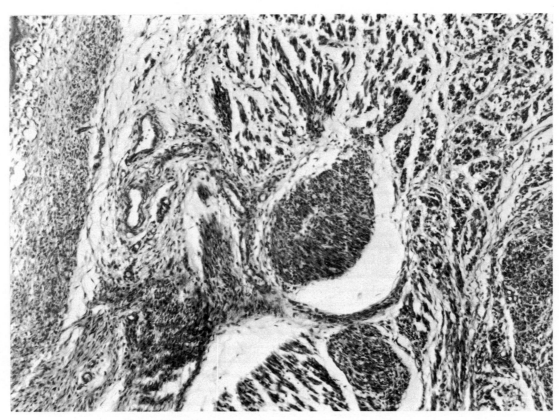

Fig. 3.101 (*series no. 1900*; neg. 14073). Level: 381. Fragment of a fourth dorsal interosseus. A connective tissue layer around the dorsal tendon is the proximal origin of the intramuscular septum. This septum is continuous with the medial fascial wall. Notice the vessels running into this membrane.

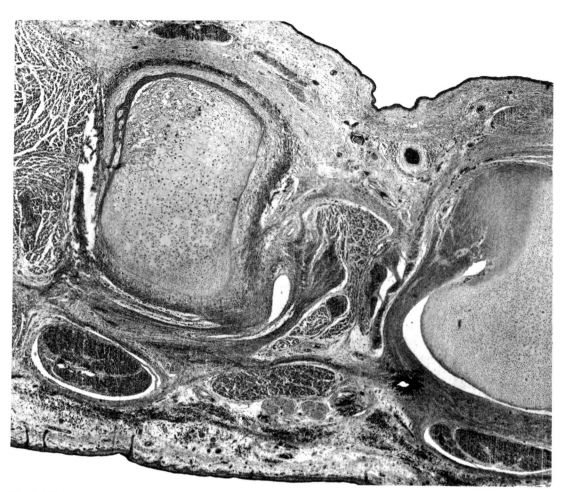

Fig. 3.102 (*series no. 1900*; neg. 14068). Level: 401. Section of the fourth intermetacarpal space. In dorsal IV we see the extension of the dorsal tendon into the volar capsule. The intramuscular septum consists of some thin fibres only. An outer layer of the dorsal tendon will delaminate to contribute to this structure. Notice the formation of a tendon fascicle on the inner side of the dorsal tendon.

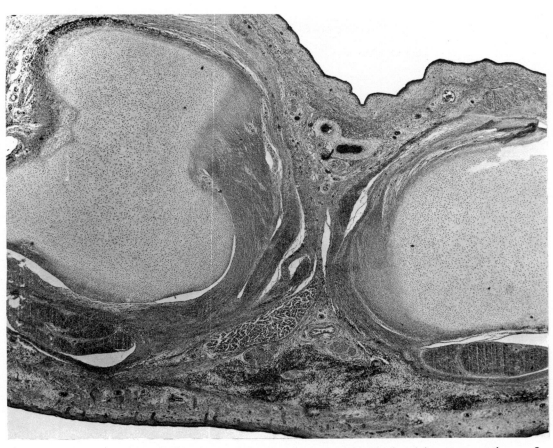

Fig. 3.103 (*series no. 1900*; neg. 14066). Level: 481. The fourth intermetacarpal space. In dorsal IV the deep tendon has been flattened in a dorsopalmar direction. Structurally it represents a double layer. The volar tendon is surrounded by a sling, the inner loop has fused entirely with the transverse lamina.

4. The Subcutaneous Hypothenar Space

This space, a most conspicuous phenomenon in cross-sections, has no counterpart on the radial side. The subcutaneous layer over the thenar eminence lacks all the typical features of the subcutaneous hypothenar space. Moreover, at proximal levels, the hypothenar space extends well over the flexor retinaculum, indeed as far as the base of the thenar eminence: and at midhand levels a relationship still exists between the subcutaneous hypothenar space and the subcutaneous midpalmar space, a relationship that does not have a corollary in the subcutaneous thenar layer. The space was investigated in transverse *series no. 1234* and *1899*.

Even in the youngest specimen, where connective tissue development is still relatively scanty, the subcutaneous hypothenar area is a conspicuous phenomenon. In the older specimen the appearance of the space is even more marked because of the dense fibrous structure of the carpal region. A dense interlacing between fascial and subcorial layers can be observed here. Both the flexor carpi ulnaris and the palmaris longus tendon reinforce the fascia with medially directed fibrous extensions. The flexor carpi ulnaris reinforces subcorial layers by direct extensions. The hypothenar space results from a division of this fibrous layer into subcorial and fascial strata. This division provides a space with a heavily reinforced subcorial roof and a reinforced fascial floor. The reinforcements are derived mainly from the flexor carpi ulnaris-pisiform column. As Figure 2.8 shows, the subcorial roof is also reinforced by anchors from the radial side, viz. from the sheath of the flexor carpi radialis. With the division of fibrous structures and the opening up of this space, the ulnar nerve and vessels are freed and come to lie in the subcutaneous space. At the same levels the fibrous layer below the ulnar nerve and vessels becomes reinforced to form the flexor retinaculum.

In *series no. 1234* the nerve and vessels are covered, for a short distance, by the inner belly of the abductor digiti V. It follows that the ulnar nerve and vessels can be approached from the subcutaneous space by rounding the inner (radial) border of the muscle (Fig. 4.6, arrow). The space extends so far over the flexor retinaculum that the palmaris longus tendon becomes located within this space. Both the subcutaneous midpalmar space and the subcutaneous hypothenar area extend from this proximal base. The spatial and structural relations within and between these regions are determined by structures such as the *palmar aponeurosis* and the *palmaris brevis* and by a number of specific fibrous skin anchorages.

Also relevant to the relations yet to be described is the formation of the ulnar flexor compartment wall in a more distal part of the mid-hand. Dissection and analysis of serial sections show the paramount importance of the anchorage to the skin. An attempt will be made by analysis of serial sections and by dissection to find out whether the often densely interwoven systems can be disentangled and made accessible.

SERIES No. 1234

Distal from the site of passage of the ramus superficialis nervi ulnaris

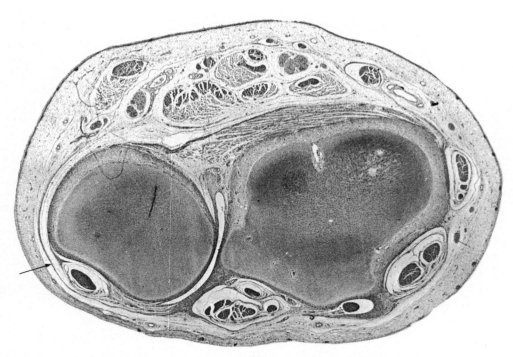

Fig. 4.1 (*series no. 1234*; neg. 10148). Section through the distal radioulnar joint. Note in particular (arrow) the superficial lamina of the fascia over the ulna and over the sheath of the extensor carpi ulnaris.

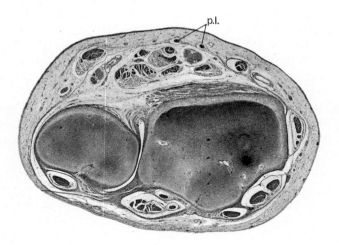

Fig. 4.2 (*series no. 1234*; neg. 4897). Section through the distal ends of radius and ulna. Note two tendons of the palmaris longus (p.l.).

and its vessels (Fig. 4.1) the fascia gains considerable strength. It extends as the ulnar and volar continuation of the extensor retinaculum surrounding the extensor carpi ulnaris sheath towards the flexor carpi ulnaris; the latter muscle reinforces this fascial lamina with strong dorsal fibrous extensions. As in more proximal sections, the superficial lamina of the fascia forms a sheath for the flexor carpi ulnaris in such a way that the fascia itself passes below the muscle, while a thin fascial covering of the flexor carpi ulnaris fuses with the underlying fascia on both sides. The flexor carpi radialis and the radial vessels run in a similar manner with the tendon in its own

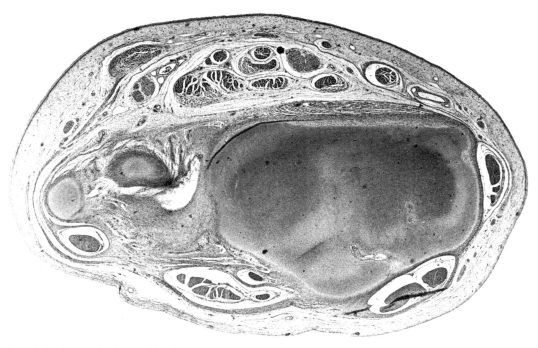

Fig. 4.3 (*series no. 1234*; neg. 10151). Section through the radiocarpal joint cleft. The strong fascial layer extending from the flexor carpi ulnaris tendon over the extensor carpi ulnaris sheath is most conspicuous.

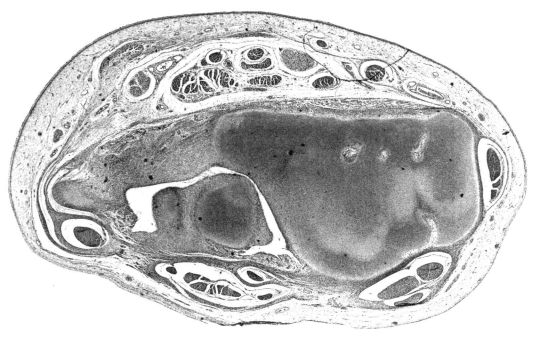

Fig. 4.4 (*series no. 1234*; neg. 10153). The lunate and triquetrum have appeared in the section.

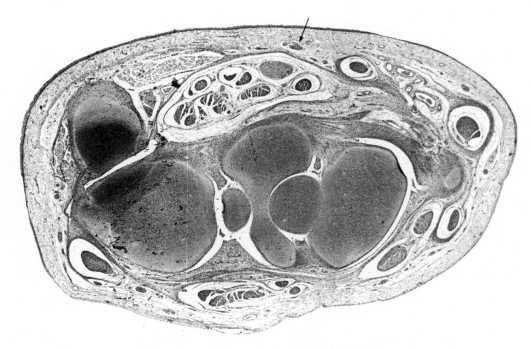

Fig. 4.5 (*series no. 1234*; neg. 10158). Section through the proximal carpal bones. The lunate is just being replaced by the capitate and hamate. The proximal base of the hypothenar subcutaneous space covers the pisiform area laterally. The palmaris longus tendon runs free over the flexor retinaculum (arrow).

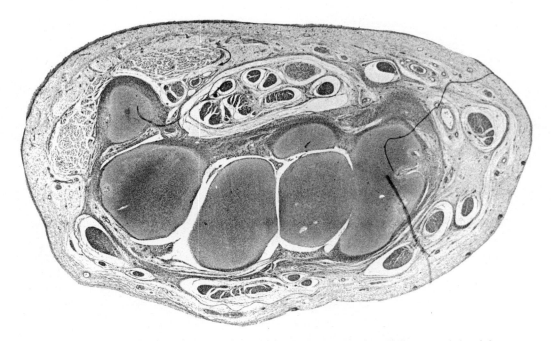

Fig. 4.6 (*series no. 1234*; neg. 10159). The space extends radially, around the abductor minimus and touches the ulnar nerve and vessels (arrow).

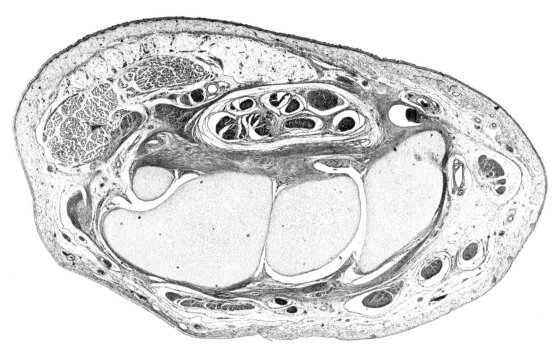

Fig. 4.7 (*series no. 1234*; neg. 4911). The pisiform area has become transformed into the pisohamate and pisometacarpal ligaments. The fascia of the hypothenar compartment is still heavily reinforced.

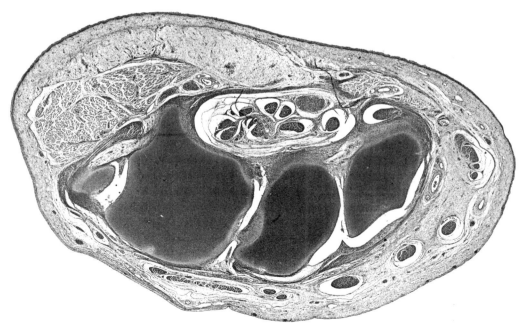

Fig. 4.8 (*series no. 1234*; neg. 4912). This figure shows a subcorial fibrous formation and the tendon of the palmaris longus in the radial part of the subcutaneous hypothenar space. Fibres from the tip of the hamulus extend over the flexor retinaculum.

sheath. Enclosed in sheaths attached to the volar fascia two tendons of the palmaris longus can be distinguished (Fig. 4.2). Through a second fascial opening, distal to that for the ulnar nerve, vessels pass from the subfascial space to the superficial subcutaneous region and vice versa. Distal to this opening a strong fibrous layer becomes apparent as the floor of the ulnar carpal region. Some breaks occur on the volar side in the continuity of the superficial lamina along the ulnar side of the ulnar palmaris longus tendon (Fig. 4.3) and these permit the passage of vessels and small nerve branches. A branch of the median nerve runs subfascially for a considerable distance before it penetrates the fascia between the flexor carpi radialis and the radial tendon of the palmaris longus (Fig. 4.4) and thus obtains an intrafascial position. The volar fascia is now gradually reinforced to produce the flexor retinaculum which passes deep to the flexor carpi radialis and the radial vessels (Fig. 4.5).

The subcutaneous hypothenar space appears at the base of the hypothenar musculature (Fig. 4.5). The proximal tip of the space is visible over the pisiform area, where we can see the flexor carpi ulnaris tendon fibres forming a cap over the cartilaginous core. The considerable reinforcement of the subcorial roof of the space by fibres of this tendon is clearly visible. The radial belly of the abductor digiti V takes origin from the fascia of the forearm by division of the layer; the muscle gradually replaces the layer. The ulnar nerve and vessels thus become located within this area and can be traced round the free radial border of the abductor digiti minimi (Fig. 4.6). The area is characterized by the development of fibrous arcades which unite its floor, which is the fibrous wall of the abductor compartment, with its roof (which is the reinforced skin at the inner side of the corium by means of a well developed fibrous layer). The main part of this area, through which the fibrous arcades run, consists of a non-fibrous cellular tissue in which the cells are arranged in a radiating fashion or in a vortex-like formation.

The pisiform area is becoming transformed into the typical cross-sections of the fibrous column from which will emerge the pisometacarpal bundles and the pisohamate ligament with its two wings. The wings run over the roof and under the floor of the flexor compartment. The bundle that runs superficial to the flexor retinaculum and in close apposition to it, gradually reinforces the ligament. The deep bundle is inserted into the base of the hamulus ossis hamati. The fibrous configuration in fact predicts the outline of the base of the bony process.

The division of the flexor retinaculum and the subcorial layers brings the palmaris longus tendon within this compartment and fibrous connections remain between the tendon and its surroundings. The tendon is attached to the wall of the radial niche in which subcorial fibres, the thenar fascia and the flexor retinaculum all meet (Fig. 4.7).

Where the palmaris longus tendon runs superficial to the flexor retinaculum, a few tiny strands become detached from the tendon which are partly lost in the subcorial formation which is seen in Figure 4.8 and these fine strands form the most proximal indication of the palmar aponeurosis: the subcorial strands detach themselves later from their subcorial position and gradually join the main

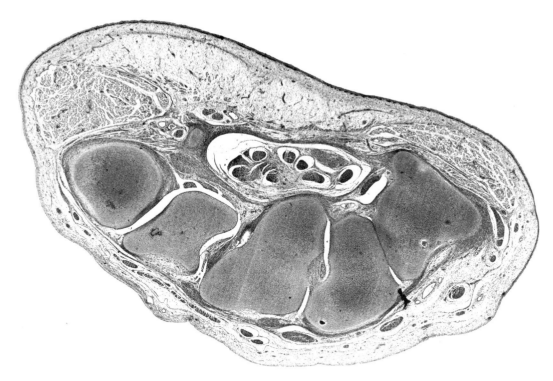

Fig. 4.9 (*series no. 1234*; neg. 10160). Section at the distal level of the hamulus. Palmaris brevis fascicles have appeared in the section. Fibres running on the inner side of the hamulus and adherent to the flexor retinaculum are seen to join the palmar aponeurosis.

palmaris longus tendon which is attached to the thenar fascia. At these levels the hamulus ossis hamati has replaced the pisohamate bundle. The pisometacarpal ligament runs along this hook and presents strong extensions towards the base of the fifth metacarpal below the gradually disappearing tendon sheath of the extensor carpi ulnaris. The tip of the hamulus serves as the site of origin of fibrous bundles that, although they are partly lost in the flexor retinaculum, maintain some of their individuality and generally run a longitudinal course. The ulnar nerve divides over the tip of the hamulus. The hypothenar fascia shows fibrous reinforcements while muscular fibres become visible in the subcutaneous space.

When the base of the fifth metacarpal widens, the insertion of the pisometacarpal bundle is seen occupying its entire palmar aspect. The two branches of the ulnar nerve and their accompanying vessels become separated from each other by a fibrous bridge between the tip of the hamulus and the abductor fascia. This fibrous bridge is soon replaced by muscular bundles that pass below the abductor to join the deep opponens, or to run distally in a superficial position. At the same levels the palmar aponeurosis has fanned out over the flexor retinaculum and a narrow space now intervenes between the two. It seems unmistakable that fascicles of the bundle running alongside the top of the hamulus and partly originating from it *leave the flexor retinacular level to join the palmar aponeurosis plane* (Fig. 4.9).

There are two conspicuous features that completely modify the

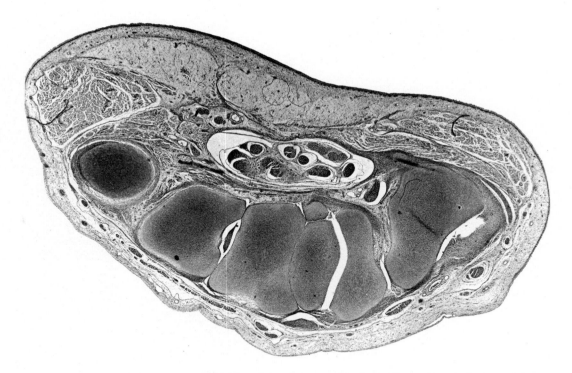

Fig. 4.10 (*series no. 1234*; neg. 10229). Section at basimetacarpal level. The superficial branches of the ulnar nerve and vessels are covered by the palmaris brevis.

picture. Firstly, the emergence of the palmaris brevis and, secondly, the gradual weakening and ultimate disappearance of the fibrous components in the palmar wall of the flexor compartment.

The origin of the palmaris brevis cannot be defined easily and precisely. There seems reasonable support, however, to say that the palmaris brevis lying in close apposition to the fascia of the abductor of the little finger originates from the niche where this fascia and the subcorial layer meet each other (Fig. 4.10). Its tendon extends into the flexor retinaculum. A most conspicuous feature visible in this section is the anchorage of the palmaris brevis system to the skin at the muscle tendon junctions of this muscle, by means of a fibrous arcade joining the tendon in a radial direction. Although the main extension of the palmaris brevis is into the flexor retinaculum, some fibres join the palmar aponeurosis layer. At the levels where the flexor retinaculum no longer extends below the ulnar vessels, its ulnar extension passes entirely into the palmaris brevis. At these levels the radial part of the ligament is seen to remain as the radial compartment wall (Fig. 4.11).

The superficial ulnar nerve has divided into its two branches. The inner branch, destined for the adjacent sides of the fourth and fifth fingers, runs now in close proximity to the parietal layer of the ulnar bursa. After the compartment wall has disappeared and also the structural relation of the opponens digiti minimi to this wall, the deep branch can pass to its deepest position. Where the flexor retinaculum does not extend as the ulnar wall of the flexor compartment an immediate communication is established between the subcutaneous

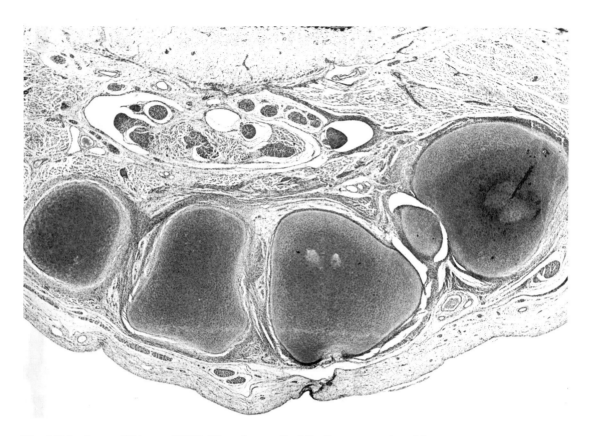

Fig. 4.11 (*series no. 1234*; neg. 10233). The palmar wall of the flexor compartment has ended. The palmaris brevis layer is the sole continuity of the radial wall of the compartment.

area and the subfascial or peritendineal space. This communication takes place around or between the fascicles of the palmaris brevis. After the palmaris brevis has left the cross-section and the palmaris longus has spread over the flexor retinaculum, a free border can be seen around which the communication takes place between the subcutaneous and subfascial spaces.

For some distance on the radial side the palmar aponeurosis remains adherent to the thenar fascia. The palmar branch of the radial artery is enclosed in this compartment below the abductor pollicis brevis, but it soon surfaces between the abductor and the opponens. The opponens fibres approach quite close to the midline in the flexor retinaculum. The radial border of the palmar aponeurosis meets the fascia at the point of enclosure of the palmar branch of the radial artery. At levels just beyond the carpus the fascial duplicature containing the palmar branch of the radial artery and its veins become accompanied by a nerve branch which emerges from the thenar muscles: this is the muscular branch of the median nerve which runs along these vessels in distoproximal direction (Fig. 4.11). Distally this nerve branch is found to be the continuation of the most palmar division of the radial branch of the median nerve. The loop of the nerve rounds the free ulnar border of the thenar eminence (Fig. 4.12). Since the continuity in the flexor compartment wall is also

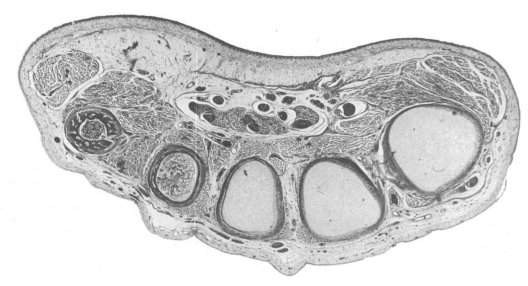

Fig. 4.12 (*series no. 1234*; neg. 25164). Section through a proximal metacarpal level. The subcutaneous hypothenar area communicates widely with the subfascial peritendineal space. The recurrent branch of the median nerve rounds the inner border of the thenar eminence.

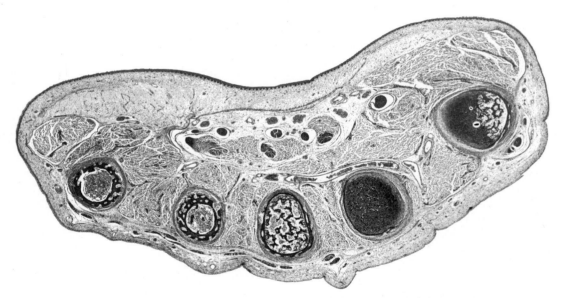

Fig. 4.13 (*series no. 1234*; neg. 12787). The palmar aponeurosis continues into subcorial strata of the thenar eminence. The ulnar compartment wall is restored by the ulnar extension of the palmar aponeurosis, in which the two layers of this structure have fused.

broken in the ulnar part of the hand the flexor retinaculum, which is now a thin fascia below the longitudinal bundles of the palmar aponeurosis, becomes somewhat suspended. The situation soon changes owing to the emergence of a subcutaneous space over the thenar eminence. A salient feature of this space is that its reinforced subcorial roof arches towards the *radial border of the palmar aponeurosis and the fascia below it,* with the result that the subcutaneous

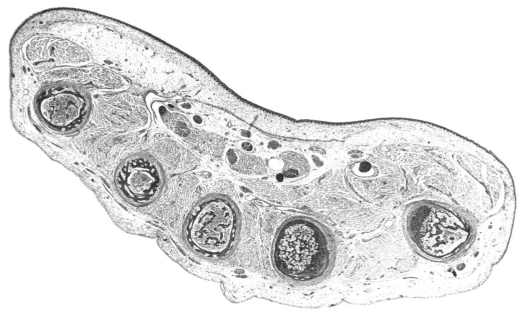

Fig. 4.14 (*series no. 1234*; neg. 25163). Section at midmetacarpal level. The grouping of the flexor tendons, lumbricals and digital nerves is well on its way.

thenar area represents a space that stands in mesenchymal continuity with the area of the long flexor tendon of the thumb (Fig. 4.14). At about the same levels, *a new ulnar compartment wall is formed*, comprising the following features: (1) the ulnar bursa is considerably narrowed as a result of the distal ending of the volar recess, (2) there is a gradual reinforcement of the ulnar bursal wall.

In addition to the reinforcement of the bursal wall proper a second wall develops around it. *This second wall is the extension of the fused palmar aponeurosis and palmar fascia*; in Figure 4.13 these two layers are seen to fuse in an ulnar direction and continue as one layer around the ulnar bursa. An areolar space or even an actual cleft intervenes between the layer derived from the palmar aponeurosis and that derived from the peritendineum of the ulnar bursa. Another further phenomenon that complicates the picture is *the anchorage of the ulnar compartment wall to the skin*. Figures 4.12 and 4.13 show fibrous strands emerging from the compartment wall and passing in a palmar direction through the subcutaneous space towards the skin. The final result is obvious, for just at levels where the subfascial space (which contains the long tendons and branches of the median and ulnar nerves) opens radially to establish an extension into the thenar area, the same space becomes closed on the ulnar side.

The observation presented so far may serve as a system of reference for observations made in a later series in which the structural picture has become more complicated as a result of continued fibrous development. This preliminary survey of the area convinced us of the need to check the ulnar and radial extensions of the palmar aponeurosis very carefully; both the layer derived from the palmaris longus and the deeper layer derived from the flexor retinaculum. The cross-sections of this stage seem to support the view that the hypothenar subcutaneous area and the thenar subcutaneous area are by no means

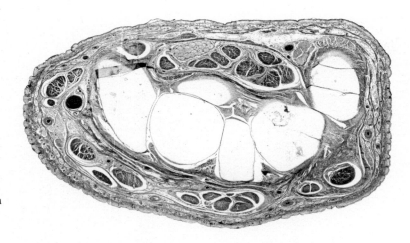

Fig. 4.15 (*series no. 1899*; neg. 15824). Level 230. Section near the proximal base of the subcutaneous hypothenar space. A dense subcorial layer is seen locally still in contact with the reinforced hypothenar fascia.

similarly or identically structured spaces. It also seems to be important to pay close attention to the proximodistal transformations taking place in the flexor carpi ulnaris-pisiform column. Finally, the relationship should be established between the course of the deep branch of the ulnar nerve and the distal end of the hamulus formation, which is also a fibrous septum.

SERIES No. 1899

Let us turn now to the observations recorded in *series no. 1899*. The analysis starts at pisiform level where the tendon of the flexor carpi ulnaris becomes transformed into the pisiform. At this level there exists a most conspicuous and characteristic anchorage of the skin to the deep fascia. Fibres extend directly into the skin overlying the pisiform and indirectly through the fascia towards subcorial layers from the flexor ulnaris tendon in both radial and distal directions. The subcutaneous hypothenar space results from separation of the fascia and subcorial layers: during this separation the fibrous bridge over the ulnar nerve and vessels disappears and this is followed by a reinforcement of the continuity of the flexor retinaculum below the ulnar nerve and vessels (Fig. 4.15). The result of all this is that the subcorial layer is seen to be heavily reinforced by longitudinal strands and to these strands the skin is attached by bundles of fibres.

The palmaris longus tendon is not primarily involved in this skin anchorage and is recognized as a separate tendon slightly adherent to the flexor retinaculum. It will be noticed that there are also some skin anchors passing from the sheath of the flexor carpi radialis in a medial direction which collectively may be called the radial skin anchor. The hypothenar space extends below this anchor and over the carpal canal where it finally touches upon the palmaris longus tendon. *At carpal levels the subcutaneous hypothenar area is marked by its strong fibrous palmar roof* (Fig. 4.16).

At these proximal levels with the pisiform still in the cross-section, muscle fibres become visible just below the subcorial layer; these fibres take their origin from connective tissue in the hypothenar area and become inserted into the radial skin anchor and they occur more or less randomly. The abductor digiti V has now appeared in the

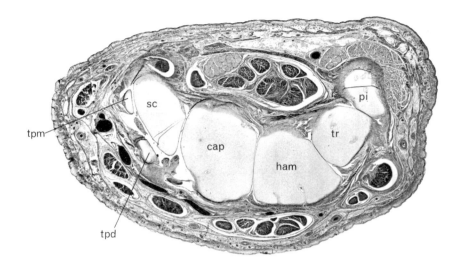

Fig. 4.16 (*series no. 1899*; neg. 16010). Level: 322. The space enlarges ulnarwards over the abductor digiti quinti. The ulnar nerve lies within the space. sc = scaphoid cap = capitate ham = hamate tr = triquetrum pi = pisiform tpm = trapezium tpd = trapezoid

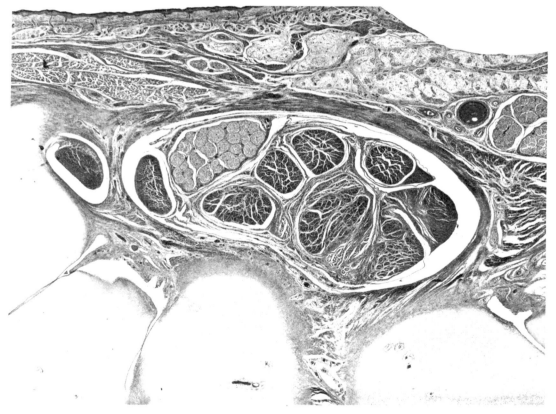

Fig. 4.17 (*series no. 1899*; neg. 13328). Level: 405. Detail of a section just proximal to the hamulus. The palmaris longus has divided into various fascicles inserted into the thenar fascia. Notice the subcorial reinforcements. The tongue-like ligament over the flexor retinaculum is perfectly clear.

cross-section with its volar compartment wall heavily reinforced by fibrous bundles from the pisiform area; the bundles are firmly anchored to the overlying skin.

The palmaris longus tendon does not remain a sharply delineated tendon for it splits into various fascicles which become anchored to

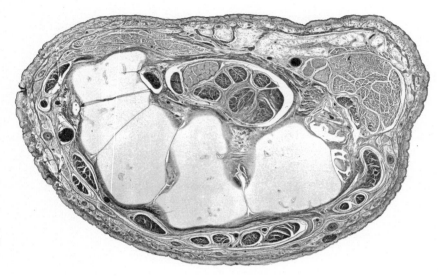

Fig. 4.18 (*series no. 1899*; neg. 16016).
Level: 434. Section through the distal
carpal bones proximal to the hamulus.
The subcorial system in the hypothenar
area in contact with the abductor fascia is
still a conspicuous feature, as is the relation
between palmar aponeurosis and subcorial
fasciculi.

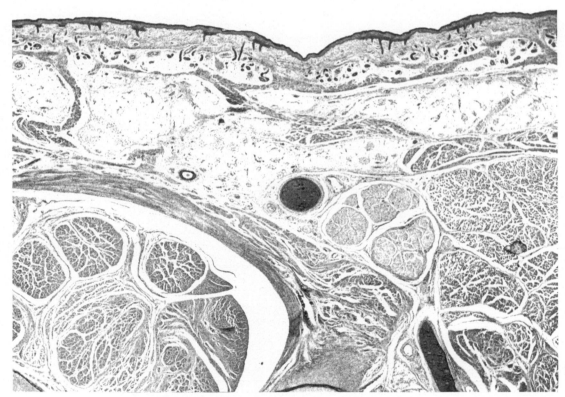

Fig. 4.19 (*series no. 1899*; neg. 18919). Level: 452. Detail of the palmaris brevis at a
proximal level becoming inserted into the subcorial layer.

the thenar compartment wall and which also establish an intimate
relationship with the subcorial system over the thenar eminence (Fig.
4.17). When thenar muscles appear in the cross-section a true radial
skin anchor ceases to exist. The twin nerves in the thenar wall
represent skin branches from the median nerve.

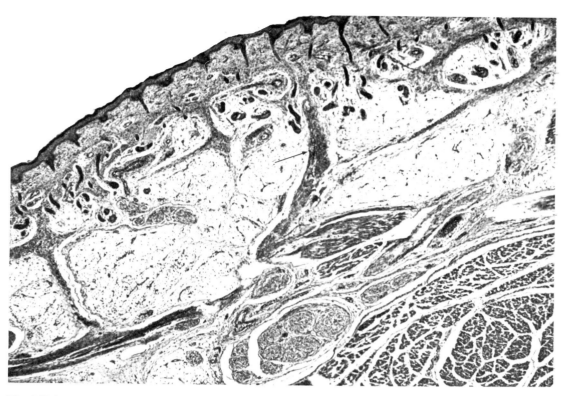

Fig. 4.28 (*series no. 1899*; neg. 18929). Level: 751. The skin anchor derived from the longitudinal bundle of Fig. 4.27 (arrow).

point where another skin anchor of the palmaris brevis is detached (Fig. 4.26). This skin anchor is a marked phenomenon. Figures 4.26 and 4.27 show a view such that one might say that the palmaris brevis tendon dichotomizes ulnarwards into the muscle layer proper and an oblique fibrous skin anchor.

Figure 4.27 clearly shows the longitudinal bundle (arrow) at the site of dichotomy. Muscle fibres are inserted into this longitudinal bundle which gives rise to a strong skin anchorage (Fig. 4.28). Gradually, however, palmaris brevis tendon fascicles curve again around the ulnar nerve to be inserted into the flexor retinaculum and the palmar aponeurosis fascicles, which were located deep to the radially inserted fibres of the palmaris brevis (Fig. 4.24), rejoin the palmar aponeurosis system. Figure 4.27 gives a clear picture of these various systems. The palmaris brevis tendon has now moved again to below the deepest palmar aponeurosis fibres and towards the thenar eminence. In this picture it is clear that the ulnar border of the palmar aponeurosis emerges from a deep position between the superficial longitudinal strands and the deepest flexor retinaculum layer. The superficial branches of the ulnar nerve gradually diverge from each other and the palmaris brevis plane is interrupted. The flexor retinaculum weakens below the ulnar nerve and its accompanying artery so that nerve and artery become in close apposition to the wall of the ulnar bursa. We see that the palmar aponeurosis is broadened by the addition of longitudinal strands, in the form of twinned fascicles, derived from a deep flexor retinaculum extension

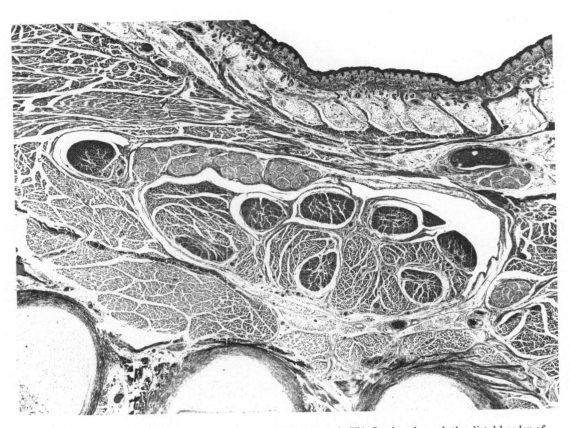

Fig. 4.29 (*series no. 1899*; neg. 13324). Level: 774. Section through the distal border of the flexor retinaculum. Notice that the most ulnar strand of the palmar aponeurosis is derived from a deep level.

(Fig. 4.29). In subsequent sections we will see that these newly added twin fascicles (Fig. 4.30, double stemmed arrow) free themselves from the palmar aponeurosis and cross a gap in the continuity of the palmaris brevis tendon. It can be seen in Figure 4.30 that this twin structure blends with the most lateral palmar aponeurosis fascicle of Figure 4.28, which has also freed itself from the palmar aponeurosis.

The twin fascicles approach a longitudinal fascicle that is still embedded in the palmaris brevis and join to form one structure (Fig. 4.31). It can be seen that this fascicle and the most lateral palmar aponeurosis fascicle are involved in one well-developed subcorial anchorage. This skin anchorage is reinforced by another lateral strand added to the palmar aponeurosis from a deeper layer (Fig. 4.32); however, the fascicles do not entirely lose their individuality and one remains visible in Figure 4.32. The distal border of the flexor retinaculum has been reached. The gap in the continuity of the palmaris brevis of Figure 4.30 is seen restored in Figure 4.32. One of the bundles in Figure 4.30 which is seen to cross the gap in the palmaris brevis plate is visible below the palmaris brevis; the other fascicles are lost in the strong oblique skin insertions of the layer (Fig. 4.32). We see also that the ulnar artery has divided into two and that the branches of the superficial nerve have diverged slightly from each other. The radial branch of the nerve flanked by the arterial branches, is in close apposition to the ulnar bursal wall, while the ulnar branch

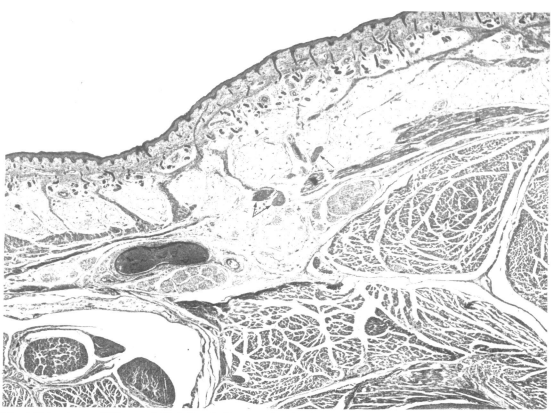

Fig. 4.30 (*series no. 1899*; neg. 18930). Level: 781. Two longitudinal fascicles derived from the palmar aponeurosis bridge the gap between aponeurosis and palmaris brevis (double arrow). In the palmaris brevis layer we still see a longitudinal bundle (arrow) derived from the anchor of Fig. 4.28. The most lateral palmar aponeurosis fascicle, the same as in Fig. 4.28, and the twin fascicle, are united in one common skin insertion.

has joined the wall of the abductor minimus. The palmaris brevis will soon disappear as a continuous layer, but before this happens we observe a remarkable phenomenon. The ulnar division of the artery is observed to divide once more into two branches, one of which circles the flexor compartment to join the deep ulnar nerve and the other becomes incorporated in the hypothenar compartment wall in a quite particular manner.

The oblique skin anchor of Figure 4.32 that is still in contact with the most lateral palmar aponeurosis fascicle by means of a subcorial system has been traced through subsequent sections, where the slope of this oblique anchor is gradually diminished and it attains a more vertical position. During this period it loses its laminar character and changes into a few strands which come into contact with the inner border of the hypothenar compartment. Still more distally the majority of these latter few strands enmesh the ulnar arterial branch into the fascial wall of the hypothenar and continue into the inner wall of the hypothenar compartment. The longitudinal bundle finds its way from below the palmaris brevis into the strands just described and thus becomes inserted into the compartment wall.

At the same time the skin anchorage of the extreme ulnar longitudinal bundle of the palmar aponeurosis (Fig. 4.32, double stemmed

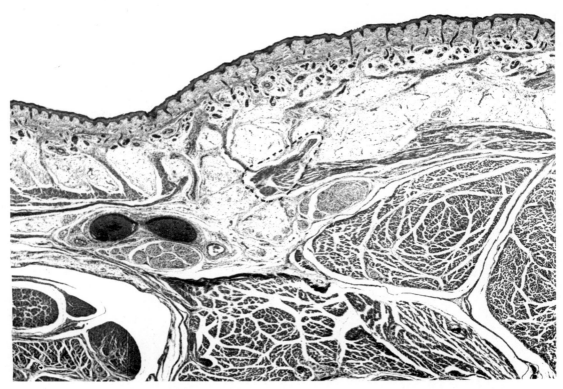

Fig. 4.31 (*series no. 1899*; neg. 18931). Level: 788. The three bundles of Fig. 4.30 have fused into one structure.

arrow) gradually loses its contact with the palmar aponeurosis and pursues its course through the subcorial layer, eventually participating in the formation of the dense fibrous structure of Figure 4.33. It is apparent that the palmaris brevis reinforces this system. It is also apparent that the oblique fibres of the palmaris brevis again extend in an ulnar direction. The most ulnar palmar aponeurosis strand in Figure 4.33 is seen to join this system (Fig. 4.34).

There are now two processes which deserve close attention: first, the closure of the flexor tendon compartment and, second, the anchorage of the ulnar compartment wall to the skin. Figure 4.34 shows that the first process is readily accomplished by an extension of the deep layer of the palmar aponeurosis and we can see that the branch of the ulnar nerve passing to the webspace between the fourth and fifth fingers is now enclosed within the compartment.

Subsequent sections show the wall to be a laminated structure and more superficial palmar aponeurosis components are likely to participate in its formation.

In the second process we see that the formation of an ulnar compartment wall establishes a continuity between the palmar aponeurosis layer and the hypothenar compartment wall, making it logical for the flexor compartment wall to continue into the septum between opponens and palmar IV. As we have seen in Figure 4.33, the inner border of the compartment wall is firmly attached to the skin and subsequent sections show that a variable number of vertical strands from subcorial strata anchor the wall to the skin (Fig. 4.35).

The most lateral palmar aponeurosis bundle in Figure 4.33 is

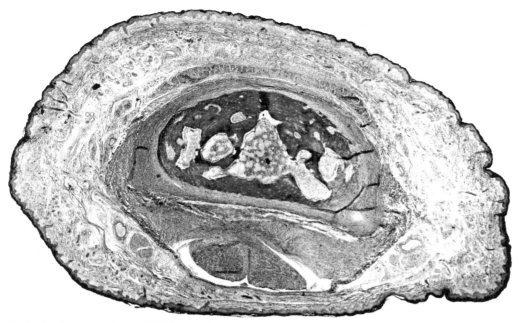

Fig. 5.7 (*series no. 1279*; neg. 21123). Level: 1759. Section through the middle phalanx close to the distal interphalangeal joint. Notice the twin structure of the profundus tendon and its contact with the volar plate.

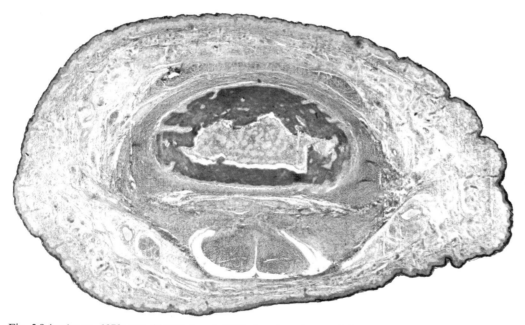

Fig. 5.8 (*series no. 1279*; neg. 21124). Level: 1744. Another picture of the proximal roots of the volar plate that form a groove for the flexor profundus tendon. Note the rich vascular bed of this tendon.

laterovolar direction, while on the palmar aspect the fibres run a frankly transverse course.

Hardly any distinction can be made between these transverse fibres and the true tendon envelope and we may say that the deepest transverse layer serves as the tendon envelope. The insertion of the

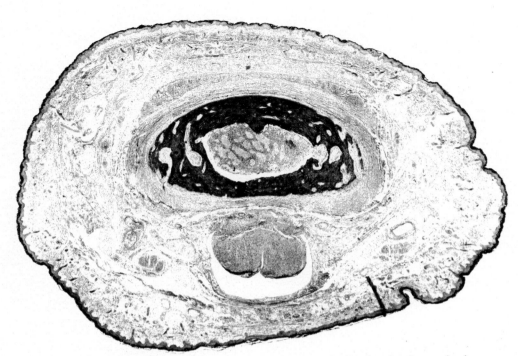

Fig. 5.9 (*series no. 1279*; neg. 21125). Level: 1675. Section showing the proximal extensions of the pillars of the volar plate which will become the fibrous tendon sheath at more proximal levels (cf. Fig. 5.10). Notice also the relation of these pillars to the skin anchorage system and the abundance of Pacinian corpuscles flanking the tendon sheath.

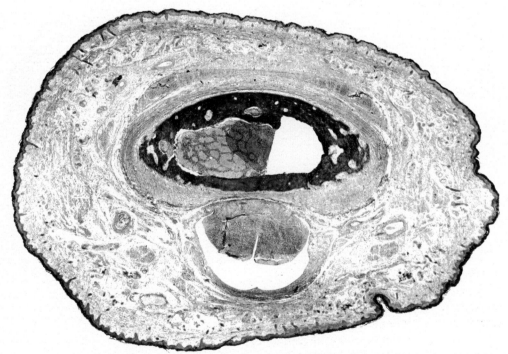

Fig. 5.10 (*series no. 1279*; neg. 21126). Level: 1644. The appearance of the strong fibrous tendon sheath. Note the extremely dense texture of the skin anchorage system.

interphalangeal ligament can be seen as soon as the skin bundles leave the bony (cartilaginous) formations of the trochlea. This ligament runs a slightly oblique dorsal course towards the middle phalanx. We also see the more volar ligaments serving as a suspension system for the volar plate. Let us now look more closely at the distal attachment of this plate. The volar margin at the base of the third phalanx becomes replaced by the volar plate of this joint. Close inspection reveals that the ligamentous mass derived from the distal phalangeal base contains a well-defined longitudinal ligament which runs on the inner side of the interphalangeal ligament and which is seen to merge with the volar plate to which the profundus tendon is still firmly adherent (Fig. 5.4). The volar plate continues over the distal phalangeal base by means of a thin layer of tissue. A capsular recess intervenes between the thick mass of this plate and the phalangeal base.

Let us now examine the situation at the phalangeal trochlea. The formation of this volar plate by ligaments originating from the middle phalanx trochlea can be seen in Figure 5.5. These ligaments are called volar accessory ligaments or volar plate ligaments and are in direct continuity with the interphalaneal ligaments. We should notice that the ligamentous layer lateral to the interphalangeal ligament which is the skin anchoring system also contributes to the volar plate and to the tendon sheath.

Subsequent sections show the proximal origin of the volar plate and the most distal extension of a synovial cleft around the profundus tendon. They also show that the strong lateropalmar anchors of the skin cease to exist and as the tendon sheath thickens so a subcutaneous layer evolves. These processes are most easily studied together. First we see the emergence of two tubercles at the lateral tips of the volar base of the trochlea, which gradually absorb the proximal lateral roots of the volar plate. In other words, the phalangeal-volar plate bundles move, with their origins, in a palmar direction along the lateral aspect of the middle phalangeal trochlea. The process can be seen in Figure 5.6 and at this same level it is noteworthy that the skin anchoring layer contributes considerably to the formation of the tendon sheath; the layer seems to restrict its skin anchorage to a system lying dorsal to the nerve-vessel bundle, but a fibrofascial sheath remains visible all round this bundle. The superficial layer of this sheath is virtually a fascial layer, while the deep layer is identical with the suspension system of the tendon sheath.

The medial portion of the volar plate thins out and simultaneously a vascular areolar tissue emerges between the plate and the bone. This vascular area is in a retroarticular or retrocapsular position. The profundus tendon which is largely surrounded by the synovial space becomes divided into two adherent fascicles which exchange fibres with the contralateral half of the volar plate (Fig. 5.7). In this same figure it is worth noting the degree to which the origin of the suspension system of the volar plate has moved to the lateropalmar tubercle. Hence the characteristic features of the proximal insertion of the volar plate are that it extends by two tongues proximally over the middle phalanx so forming a bed for the tendon of the flexor profundus (Fig. 5.8) and that the tongues are suspended laterally from the laterobasal side of the trochlea. The middle portion of the volar plate thins out considerably and it becomes replaced by vascular tissue rich in Pacinian corpuscles. It is remarkable that the fibrous tongues continue to radiate fibres into the skin in dorsolateral directions. There are hardly any longitudinally running fibres to be seen in the midlateral plane of the finger, even dorsal to the nerve-vessel bundle, in a plane that at a previous level (Fig. 5.6) was still dense with transverse fibrous tufts. At the levels under consideration a conspicuous fibrous transformation occurs, in a proximal direction, in the tubercles on the basal aspect of the middle trochlea. These areas will give rise to the fascicles of the sublimis tendon. On cross-section the triangular shaped halves of the volar plate become progressively thinner as seen in Figure 5.8. At a certain level they lose their connection with the laterobasal aspect of the trochlea, *which means that the retrocapsular area, which has now become a subtendinous area, is made accessible from outside the tendon sheath area.* The triangular masses, i.e. the proximal tongues of the volar plate, become transformed into club-shaped thickenings at the dorsal tips of a tendon sheath in a quasi-suspended position (Fig. 5.9). The volar part of the tendon sheath thickens as the two tongues of the volar plate become absorbed into the sheath. Figures 5.8 to 5.11 show how this probably occurs.

Thus it seems that the middle phalangeal osteofibrous segment of the tendon sheath is a continuity of the volar plate and of the tendon sheath at distal interphalangeal level; when viewed from a proximo-distal direction the tendon sheath is anchored to the volar plate by two pillars. Particularly notable is the broad access to the vascular bed of the flexor profundus along the basal side of the phalanx, a route containing many Pacinian bodies.

Extensions from the sheath proper which pass deep to the volar nerve and artery and from overlying layers which pass superficial to the volar nerve and vessels, find their way into the skin anchoring system. There are conspicuous dense longitudinal strands cut transversely which run dorsal to the nerve-vessel sheath; it should be noted that these strands detach proximally from subcorial layers and hence they are not a *direct* continuation of strands originating from the distal joint.

We arrive at levels now where the terminal tendon starts dividing into two fascicles and at which the tendon sheath again closes entirely around the flexor tendon and its vascular bed; within the sheath lie *also the proximal extensions of the palmar tubercles of the trochlea and these appear to become transformed into the two fascicles of the flexor sublimis* (Figs. 5.10 and 5.11).

The sheath itself becomes directly continuous with the thick periosteal layer of the middle phalanx, a situation which anticipates the adult state in which the sheath forms an osteofibrous compartment containing the bone. As can be seen in dissections it is typical of the formation of the sheath that it does not become inserted into a bony crest but continues around the bone as a thick periosteal investment.

We see also the development of an areolar space between the flexor tendon sheath and the overlying fascia with both structures continuing to contribute to the skin anchoring system. Another feature that cannot be missed and that plays an important role in the arrangement of the proximal interphalangeal region is seen in the terminal tendon when it becomes enveloped in a fold of tissue derived from the fascial layer that surrounds the flexor tendon sheath. This fascia also envelops the nerve and artery and becomes increasingly noticeable at the levels under consideration. Dorsal to the vessels, the fascial envelope merges with the anchoring system of the skin which becomes considerably denser at these levels. It is obvious that those tendons which make up the sublimis will become isolated from the floor of the tendon sheath and the adjoining walls, a process which coincides with considerable thinning of the fibrous wall of the tendon compartment.

While the fascicles of the sublimis are still situated in the lateral niches of the sheath, this sheath appears to end with a free proximal border while it is being replaced by a more fascial sheath derived from the emerging suspension system (Fig. 5.12). This section provides the relevant evidence as it shows the sickle-like remnants of the free proximal border of the middle phalangeal osteofibrous segment of the sheath. The emergence of another segment of the tendon sheath, suspended from the phalangeal base, coincides with a similar change in the arrangement of the digital fascia. This fascia also obtains a strong anchorage to the periosteum of the middle phalanx precisely at those levels where the thick periosteal investment derived from the osteofibrous tendon sheath is becoming thinner. A suspension system emerges for both the fascia and the *proximal interphalangeal segment* of the tendon sheath. The digital fascia encloses the nerve and artery. An extremely conspicuous skin anchorage system becomes apparent at those levels which are approaching the proximal interphalangeal joint. Figure 5.12 illustrates this point very nicely. Extremely dense bundles of fibres are seen here between the lateral aspect of the bone and the skin. The subcorial thickening in the lateral aspect of the skin is equally impressive. It seems beyond doubt that this skin anchorage system blends with the suspension system above mentioned.

This arrangement makes it quite logical that this skin anchorage system should extend proximally over the ligament layer of the proximal interphalangeal joint to be inserted into the trochlear region of the proximal phalanx. We have to look closely at this situation in the proximal interphalangeal joint because of the presence of the retinacular system that covers the lateral aspect of the joint, so preventing to some extent a lateral approach from the exterior. As we approach the joint, the skin anchorage system seems to become more laminar (Fig. 5.13).

We cannot escape noticing how very different are the two sides of the section from each other. There is obviously some obliquity in the plane of section but this could hardly account for differences of this magnitude. It is more probable that irregular compression of the section combined with exaggeration of the extensions has produced this unusual picture. This does not prevent us from establishing that towards the proximal interphalangeal joint the fascia which enfolds the nerve-vessel bundles becomes suspended from the base of the middle phalanx and is joined by the anchorage system. A deep layer of this suspension fascia continues into the proximal interphalangeal segment of the sheath and the volar plate. We are reminded of the pattern of the terminal tendon as it lies enclosed in the fascial

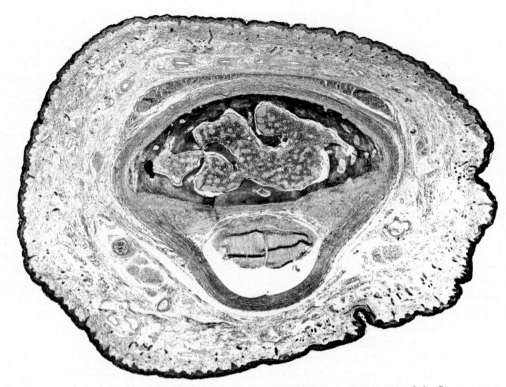

Fig. 5.11 (*series no. 1279*; neg. 21128). Level: 1591. The distal roots of the flexor sublimis are confined within the flexor tendon sheath. The fascial envelope around the terminal tendon has become more marked. Note the areolar space around the tendon sheath and the strong development of the skin anchorage system and its relations.

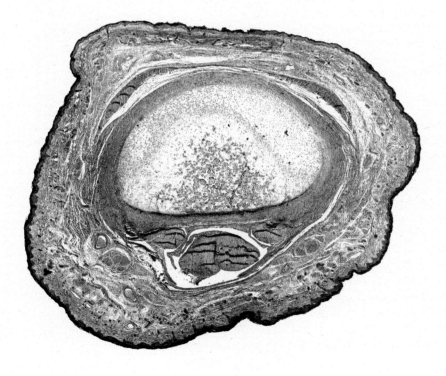

Fig. 5.12 (*series no. 1279*; neg. 22504). Level: 1480. Section through the middle phalanx at the proximal border of the tendon sheath of phalanx II.

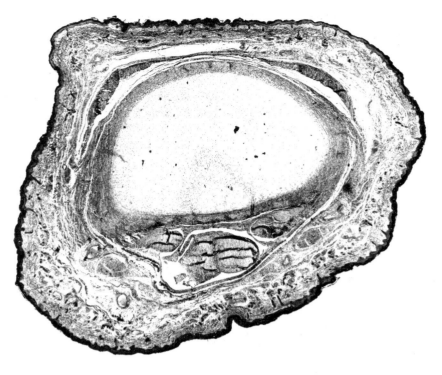

Fig. 5.13 (*series no. 1279*; neg. 20473). Level: 1461. Section near the base of the second phalanx. The digital fascia represents a layer of the suspension system which will soon involve the tendon sheath and volar plate. Notice at the radial (left) side of this section the extremely dense fibrous laminae, partly skirting the volar border of the terminal tendon and lying between the lateral skin and the phalanx.

duplicature derived from the volar fascia, which allows terminal tendon fibres to merge with these fascial structures, while the free lateral border of the terminal tendon becomes more or less buried in this fascial layer.

Approaching the proximal interphalangeal joint we see the pattern described above merge with the ligamentous structures of the joint. The thick fibrous investment of the base of the phalanx gives rise to the middle tendon of the extensor assembly, the volar plate, the interphalangeal ligaments and a fascial layer covering the fibrous tendon sheath. This situation is similar to the one seen in the distal interphalangeal joint, in so far as in both joints the interphalangeal ligament is surrounded by a thick fibrous system. In the distal joint this system is mainly a skin anchorage system, while in the proximal joint, the volar plate and tendon sheath are suspended from the base of the phalanx and from the trochlea of the proximal phalanx by this same system. From the tendon sheath we see that fibres radiate laterally towards the skin. The skin anchors of the middle segment of the finger were seen to merge with pericapsular fibrous layers, a point that needs verifying by micro-dissection. Another result of the blending of the digital fascia with the sheath proper is that the sheath itself becomes part of the neurovascular sheath.

Both the volar extension of the extensor assembly and the anchorage of a transverse retinacular ligament into the tendon sheath are features in Figures 5.14 and 5.15. These sections pass through the joint and they show the massive ligamentous origins from the trochlea of the first phalanx. Each ligamentous area comprises the interphalangeal ligament and the suspension system around it. It is evident that the ligaments situated in the same stratum as the

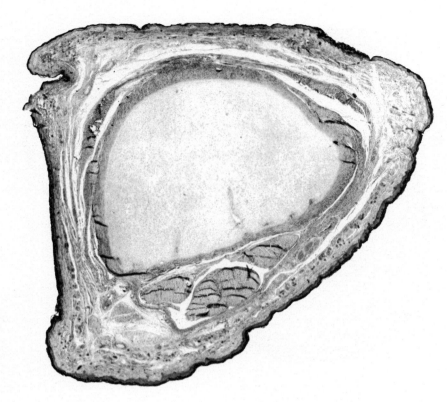

Fig. 5.14 (*series no. 1279*; neg. 21129).
Level: 1389. Section through the middle
phalanx. A fascial sheet has developed
between the sublimis fascicles. The tendon
sheath layer extends dorsally as a thick
periosteum, as far as the area indicating
the insertion of the middle tendon. The
continuity of the terminal tendon layer
with volar structures is most conspicuous.

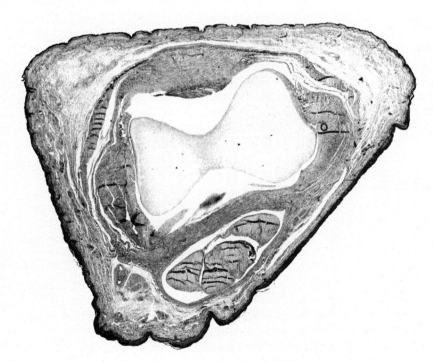

Fig. 5.15 (*series no. 1279*; neg. 21130).
Level: 1315. Section through the distal tip
of the trochlea of the first phalanx. The
interphalangeal bundle is not yet inserted
into the bone. Bundles are visible from the
bone skirting the former, on their way
towards the volar plate and the tendon
sheath. Notice also the situation of the
lateral border of the extensor assembly.
○ = interphalangeal ligament.

interphalangeal layer but in a more palmar position also belong to
the suspension system (Fig. 5.17).

The configuration of the trochlea of the first phalanx is extremely
characteristic, viz. the trapezoid shape on cross-section, the position
of the three fascicles (or tendons) of the extensor assembly and the

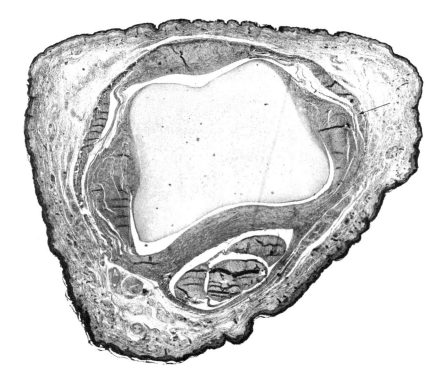

Fig. 5.16 (*series no. 1279*; neg. 21131).
Level: 1280. Section through the core of
the trochlea of the first phalanx.
Conspicuous features are the thick volar
plate, the ligaments originating from the
trochlea, the interphalangeal and the
phalangeal-glenoidal ligament; the latter
also contributes to the tendon sheath.
The position of fascicles of the extensor
assembly is also typical. arrow=oblique
part of retinacular ligament.

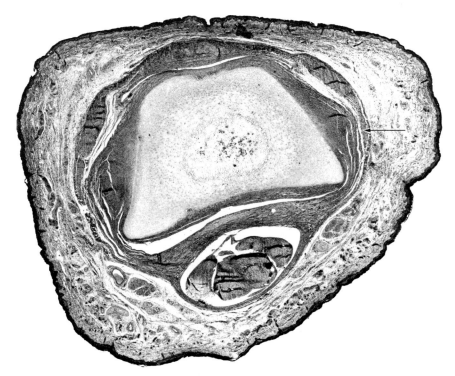

Fig. 5.17 (*series no. 1279*; neg. 21132).
Level: 1225. A section closer to the
proximal insertion of the volar plate.
Notice the heavy development of
ligaments to the volar plate and to the
tendon sheath which are derived from the
trochlea. The arrow points to the oblique
part of the retinacular ligament.

palmar extension of the extensor assembly layer. Longitudinal fibres
are seen to assemble at the palmar tip of the lateral band of the
extensor assembly forming an oval-shaped tendon which adds a new
lateral border to the extensor assembly (Fig. 5.17). This oval-shaped
tendon or oblique part of the retinacular ligament will be traced to

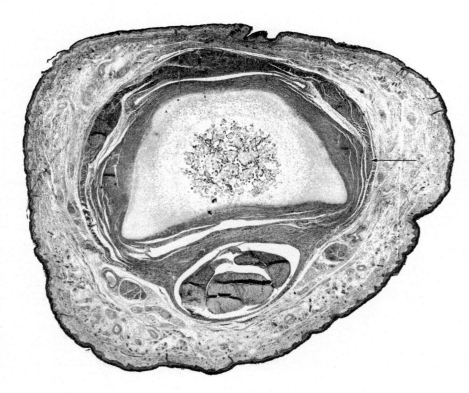

Fig. 5.18 (*series no. 1279*; neg. 21133).
Level: 1208. The ligaments anchoring the
volar plate have now reached the basal
tubercles of the trochlea. arrow=oblique
part of retinacular ligament.

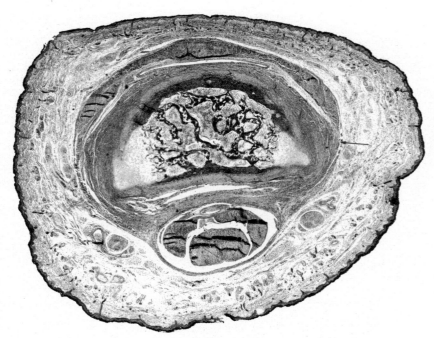

Fig. 5.19 (series no. *1279*; neg. 21134).
Level: 1165. The proximal capsular recess
of the joint is now cut. Notice the position
of the oblique band within a fascial layer
(arrow).

its insertion into the shaft of the proximal phalanx, close to the distal
exit of the proximal phalangeal segment of the tendon sheath (Fig.
5.23). Further observations relevant to this system will be presented
subsequently.

Let us first describe the sheath at the proximal interphalangeal
level and the volar plate in more detail. For detail of the distal

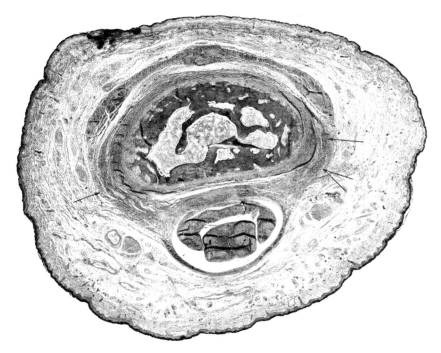

Fig. 5.20 (*series no. 1279*; neg. 21135). Level: 1114. Section through the first phalanx with the volar plate in the process of becoming inserted. Notice the bundles in close connection to the phalanx (cf. Figs. 5.18 and 5.19). arrows=oblique ligaments; double stemmed arrow= anchors of volar plate.

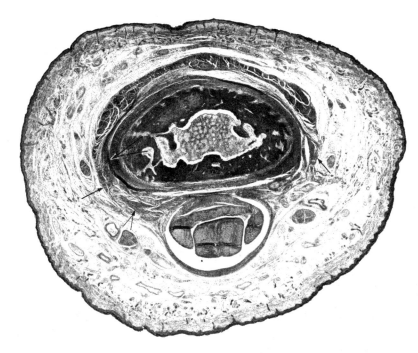

Fig. 5.21 (*series no. 1279*; neg. 21888). Level: 1086. Section through the vascular hilum proximal to the proximal interphalangeal joint. One of the proximal roots of the volar plate is located in a juxta-trochlear position, the other one in a more basal position. The oblique bands are in close apposition to the roots of the volar plate. There is a considerable thickening in the volar part of the sheath that will also shift dorsally in more proximal sections (cf. Fig. 5.23). arrows= oblique bands; double stemmed arrows= roots of volar plate.

insertion of the volar plate and the formation of a capsular recess between plate and phalangeal base, we refer the reader to the sagittal series; here it suffices to point out the strongly anchored suspension system from which the plate is derived (Fig. 5.14). It seems, moreover, that volar plate and phalangeal base are most intimately linked across the entire width of the phalangeal base. The volar plate is fully developed in Figure 5.15 and the tendon sheath is seen to be still only moderately thick. The situation is maintained through Figures 5.16

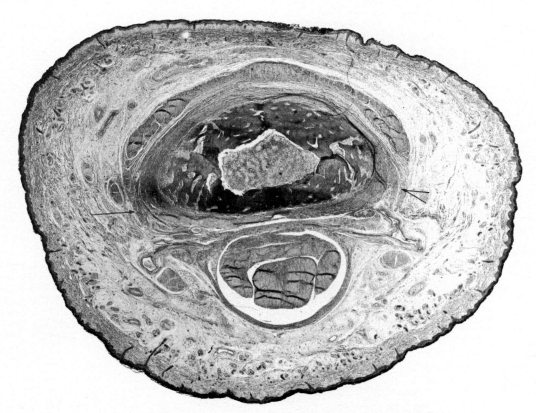

Fig. 5.22 (*series no.* 1279; neg. 21136). Level: 1055. A dense contribution of vessels to the vascular bed of the sublimis. The bundles, marked by a double stemmed arrow, represent the oblique band and a proximal anchor of the sheath or volar plate. They are now almost fully inserted into the phalangeal shaft close to the volar lateral borders. arrow = oblique band; double stemmed arrow = fused oblique band and anchor.

and 5.17, while in 5.18 and 5.19 the tendon sheath itself appears to thin out to such a degree that no more than a fascial hood remains around the tendons. All the figures mentioned provide ample evidence for the suspension of the volar plate in so far as the suspension ligaments cover the interphalangeal ligaments on their lateral aspects, while a significant contribution to the volar plate is derived from fibres belonging to the same layer as the interphalangeal ligaments.

Figure 5.19 shows the roots of the ligaments derived from the trochlea which contribute to the volar plate in this way.
As can be seen in this figure the area of origin is not confined to a circumscribed place on the lateral aspect of the trochlea, but the origin of these ligaments extends right to the palmar border of the lateral trochlear surface.

We are approaching those levels at which the proximal insertion of the volar plate will occur. At the levels we will be passing (Figs. 5.20 up to and including 5.25) we will see the emergence of a new reinforcement strip in the tendon sheath, a reinforcement which seems to arise bilaterally from the volar plate (Figs. 5.19 and 5.20) and which later removes bilaterally in a dorsal direction; this is most impressive in Figure 5.23. At levels between Figures 5.20 and 5.23 the system forms a considerable palmar reinforcement. It is obvious that

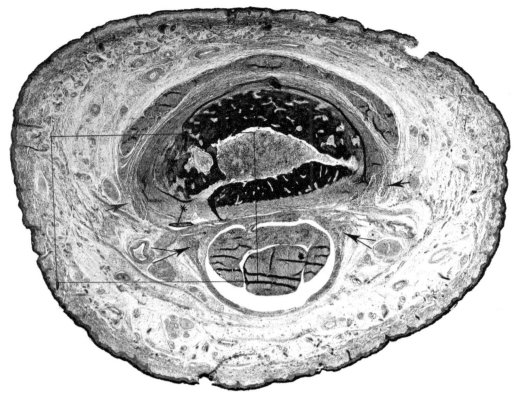

Fig. 5.23 (*series no. 1279*; neg. 21137). Level: 1031. Section through the proximal phalanx proximal to the crossing of the cruciate ligaments. The proximal extensions of the oblique parts of the retinacular ligaments. The club-shaped extensions of the volar plate are well visible (double stemmed arrows). *=one of the proximal roots of the volar plate; arrows=oblique ligaments.

here we now see the so-called cruciate ligaments of the tendon sheath.

Let us look at what is happening to the volar plate. A figure such as 5.19 shows clearly the lateral anchorage of the volar plate, an anchorage that extends right to the basal border of the lateral side of the trochlea. We see in Figure 5.20 that while this strictly lateral anchoring system is ending, a few discrete anchoring bundles extend proximally from the volar plate. One bundle is seen just below the oblique band mentioned earlier, with which it runs along the lateral ridge of the phalanx in a proximal direction (Fig. 5.20). Another bundle is found nearer the basal side of the phalanx and more in line with the lateral border of the tendon sheath; it is shown in Figure 5.21 and as a hilum develops when the lateral volar plate suspension anchors end, we see that this bundle runs amidst vessels and nerves which pass through this hilum to the retroarticular, subtendineal, vascular areas of the proximal interphalangeal joint. We should look now at what has happened in the meantime to the other component of the complex, viz. the sheath itself. We should recall here that the cruciate system, obviously derived from the volar plate, returns in a laterodorsal direction after becoming crossed.

In the meantime the volar plate has disappeared and these ligaments now appear as club-like swellings of a tendon sheath in a quasi-suspended position (Fig. 5.23). Later and proximal to the vascular

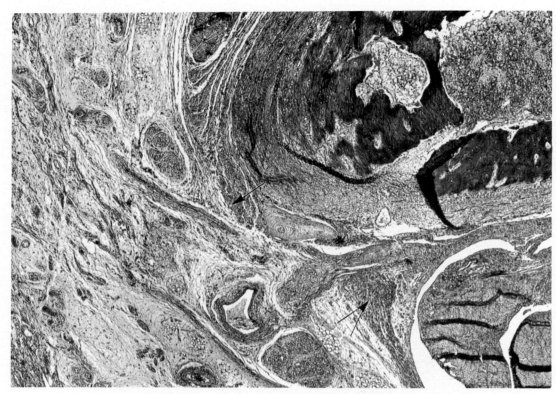

Fig. 5.24 (*series no. 1279*; neg. 21137). Level: 1031. Detail of the rectangle of Fig. 5.23. The proximal extension of the retinacular ligament and of one of the proximal roots of the volar plate are visible. Notice the club-like swelling at the dorsal tip of the sheath (double stemmed arrow). *=one of the proximal roots of the volar plate; arrow=oblique ligament.

Fig. 5.25 (*series no. 1279*; neg. 14578). Level: 998. Section just distal to the osteofibrous sheath of phalanx I. The extremely dense fibrous areas at the insertion of the sheath into the phalanx at this level are very conspicuous just proximal to the vascular hilum. The oblique retinacular ligament (arrow), the most proximal roots of the volar plate and the cruciate ligaments of the sheath proper are found in this area. The fairly dense concentrations related to the skin anchoring system are also noteworthy.

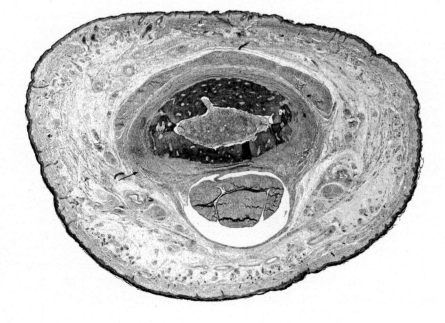

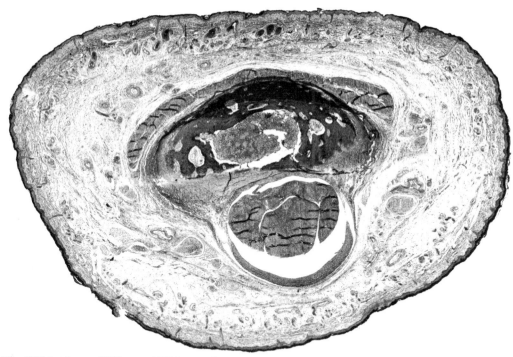

Fig. 5.26 (*series no. 1279*; neg. 21138). Level: 984. The sickle indicating the distal border of the osteofibrous section of the sheath of phalanx I. This sickle is located within the fascial reinforcement of the sheath at proximal interphalangeal level.

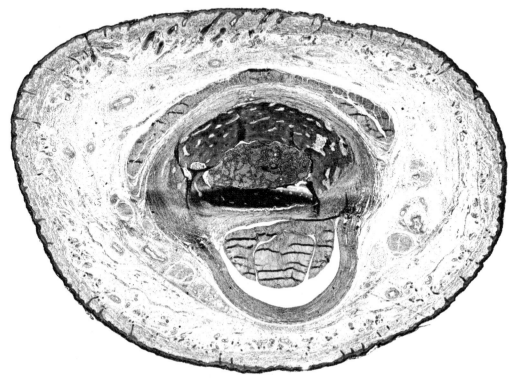

Fig. 5.27 (*series no. 1279*; neg. 21139). Level: 942. A typical cross-section at midphalangeal level. The extremely strong tendon sheath is the most marked feature. Notice also the strong development of the digital fascia in front of the sheath and its role in the formation of the nerve-vessel sheath as well as its contribution to the digital band.

hilum the longitudinal fibrous strands or anchors derived from the volar plate become inserted into a fairly thick fibrous area at the lateral border of the volar aspect of the phalanx (Fig. 5.25). It is clear that these fibrous areas also hold the proximal roots of the cruciate ligaments of the sheath.

The fibrous sickle that heralds the osteofibrous sheath of phalanx I will soon develop within the extremely thin tendon envelope (Fig. 5.26). This segment of the sheath becomes firmly inserted into the phalanx and then becomes surrounded by an areolar cleft which separates it from the somewhat reinforced digital fascia.

In Figure 5.27 it is important to decide whether or not this areolar space is identical to the space around the tendon sheath of the proximal interphalangeal level or if it represents the space in Figure 5.26, which seems to be present between the fibrous sickle and the fascial remnant of the interphalangeal sheath section. Careful screening of the relevant sections leads us to the conclusion that an extremely attenuated proximal extension of the proximal interphalangeal sheath section eventually becomes attached to the tendon sheath. This would mean that if the areolar space of Figure 5.27 is followed distally it would lead over the sheath, although the space itself has narrowed considerably.

It is rewarding to pay some attention to this situation and to compare it with the situation found in the distal interphalangeal joint. We recall that a marked retroarticular vascular area was seen in this joint, that the volar plate with its roots could be followed proximally and instead of being inserted into the phalanx it *merged with the middle phalangeal osteofibrous part of the tendon sheath*. Therefore, in the distal joint the proximal extensions of the volar plate are seen to pass primarily into the tendon sheath and only secondarily into the middle phalangeal shaft; in the proximal joint these roots are inserted into the shaft immediately proximal to the retroarticular vascular area. The tendon sheath of the first phalanx arises independently from the most proximal anchors of the volar plate and it seems that this feature is a point of fundamental difference between these two joints.

Some further observations relevant to the retinacular system will be presented now. Figures 5.16 to 5.19 show a fibrofascial continuity of the extensor assembly into the flexor tendon sheath. These volar extensions overlie the fibrous suspension layer of the volar plate. The fibrofascial extensions are continuous distally with the digital fascia, in which the vessels are embedded (Fig. 5.14). Proximally this fascia gradually merges with the sheath so that the sheath itself becomes the inner wall of the nerve-vessel sheath (Figs. 5.16 and 5.17). In its turn the tendon sheath sends fibres to the skin in a dorsolateral direction. Passing proximally within this palmar fascial radiation we soon notice that the extensor assembly acquires a thickened knob-like lateral border located just on the palmar side of an imaginary line dividing the trochlea into dorsal and volar halves.

It is not easy to trace accurately the origin of these fibres in the terminal tendon. The impression is gained that they seem to form a cord from dorsal fibres in the terminal tendon; the tendinous cord-like free border is found within the volar fascial extensions and it cannot be defined very sharply. As Figure 5.18 shows, the volar knob

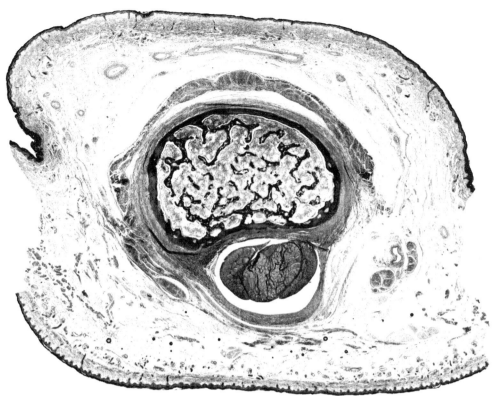

Fig. 5.28 (*series no. 1279*; neg. 21140). Level: 754. A section passing distally through the natatorial fold. Marked reinforcement of the digital fascia, junctions with the natatorial ligament and longitudinal fibres of the latter system in the fold can all be seen.

is much more noticeable on the ulnar than the radial side, certainly at this level. On following this tendinous cord in a proximal direction we see that it becomes juxtaposed to the suspension ligaments. It would also seem that this cord gives its own extensions volarwards which merge with the volar extensions of the suspension ligament. Although the cord never loses its individuality it is difficult and even impossible to define it accurately in deeper layers.

Figures 5.20 and 5.21 show the oblique bands in close apposition to the most lateral anchor of the volar plate to the proximal phalanx. The anchors are soon lost in the periosteal layers, but proximally, the oblique bands remain discernable as such, as do the anchors of the volar plate, which are located more towards the palmar side (Fig. 5.21). The close relationship between the ligaments mentioned and the skin anchorage system is worthy of note as it becomes conspicuous at these levels.

In this way the vascular hilum of the retroarticular bed is bordered by the oblique band of the retinacular ligament dorsally and by the most proximal anchor of the volar plate ventrally. We can be sure therefore that two extremely rich vascular supplies pass to the contents of the sheath; one passes between the distal interphalangeal joint and the middle phalangeal osteofibrous portion of the tendon sheath while the other passes proximal to the proximal interphalangeal joint and distal to the reinforced part of the sheath related to the shaft of the first phalanx.

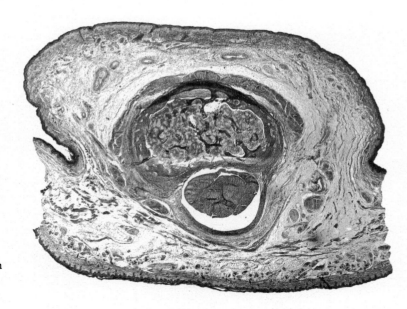

Fig. 5.29 (*series no. 1279*; neg. 21674). Level: 700. Fibrous structures are seen in the natatorial fold. Marked dorsal radiations are present from the phalanx.

Seen as it lies along the shaft of the first phalanx the tendon sheath seems to be a rather autonomous structure. A view as seen in Figure 5.26 suggests that the sheath emerges as an individual structure within the sheath at more distal levels. Proximally the two segments of the sheath then fuse and the space between them is obliterated. An areolar space around the sheath becomes more marked (Fig. 5.27) than at articular and retroarticular levels, as a result of fascial laminations emerging to re-establish a true digital fascia enclosing the nerve-vessel bundle.

The situation anticipates a strong reinforcement of this digital fascia into a hood which has a fibrous texture and which will replace the tendon sheath segment of the proximal phalanx.

Figure 5.26 represents a typical cross-section at the proximal phalangeal level. In addition to our earlier findings regarding the tendon sheath and its fascial covering we see here a gradual segregation into separate bundles of the extensor and interosseous (or lumbrical) tendon fibres. We also see a gradual thinning of the layer between the sublimis fascicles.

While the digital fascia is decidedly at a deeper level than the subcorial system, interconnections occur frequently between the two. Towards the natatorial fold the increase in density in the fascial hood becomes more and more marked.

The basal digital fold itself as might be expected is the site of most impressive fibrous condensations. Quite a few of the fibres giving rise to this dense tissue take on a longitudinal course and can be followed in subsequent sections of the webspace (Figs. 5.28 and 5.29). We will comment upon them more extensively later. It should be noted that in the lateral line of the finger quite a few longitudinal fibres are cut which intercross with a system radiating from the lateral aspect of the tendon sheath and from the fascial hood over it and from the basal aspect of the phalanx.

A glance at a section such as the one shown in Figure 5.28 allows us to see the increasing thickness of the fascial hood around the tendon sheath and also the condensed fibrous system lying over this

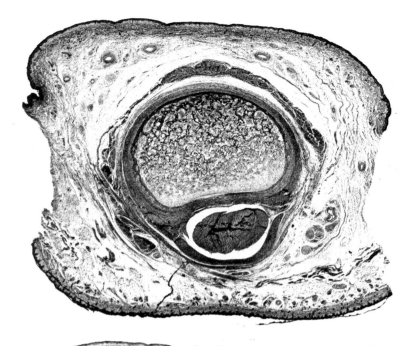

Fig. 5.30 (*series no. 1279*; neg. 21673). Level: 655. This figure shows structural continuities between the natatorial system, the fascial hood over the tendon sheath, the nerve-vessel sheath and dorsal subcutaneous layers.

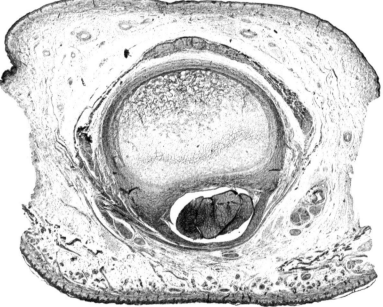

Fig. 5.31 (*series no. 1279*; neg. 21672). Level: 634. The nerve-vessel sheath at the root of the finger. The natatorial system is visible in both webspaces. Radiations passing towards the dorsal fold through the medium of the nerve-vessel sheath can be seen.

hood and the numerous interconnections; this fibrous system is the natatorial ligament which in its turn becomes connected with subcorial strata.

As mentioned earlier, an interesting feature is the extremely dense concentration of tissue lateral to the phalanx, from which site fibres radiate into the dorsal interdigital fold. The longitudinal transversely-cut fibres in the fold proper should not be overlooked; some of them pass into the finger along the line extending from this fold instead of becoming inserted into the interdigital fold and hence they are in a more volar position than those longitudinal fibres found between the lateral aspect of the phalanx and the skin.

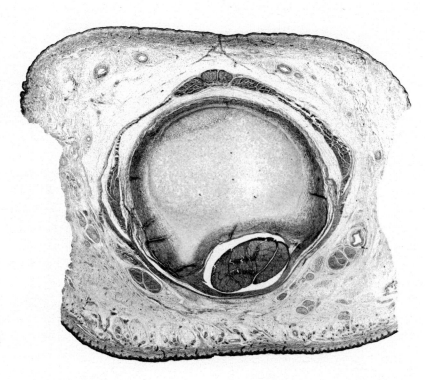

Fig. 5.32 (*series no. 1279*; neg. 21889).
Level: 593. Section through the phalangeal
base, close to the proximal end of the
tendon sheath of phalanx I.

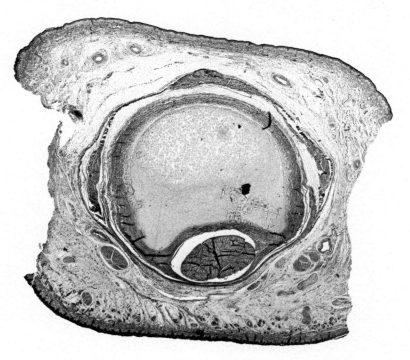

Fig. 5.33 (*series no. 1279*; neg. 21671).
Level: 573. The tendon sheath of phalanx
I is relatively thin. The fibrous hood over
it represents the digital fascia (cf. Figs.
5.29 and 5.30).

Continuities (or anchorages) are established between the skin and
the shaft of the phalanx by means of exfoliations of the natatorial
system into the skin and interconnections between the natatorial
system and the fascial hood. Proximally it is striking that the longitudinal bundles in the natatorial fold subsist for a time and that the
two layers around the tendon sheath tend to remain separate from

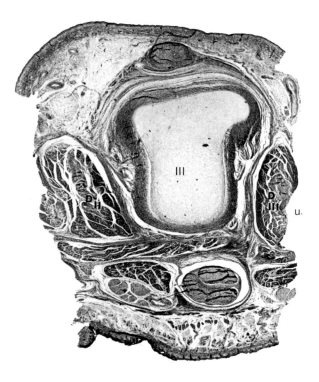

Fig. 5.56 (*series no. 1279*; neg. 21652). Level: 122. Longitudinal bundles in the partitions of the palmar aponeurosis. A fibrous layer lies between the interosseous and the metacarpal shaft and a fibrous interosseous compartment is formed. r. = radial; u. = ulnar; D II = dorsal II; III = metacarpal III; D III = dorsal III.

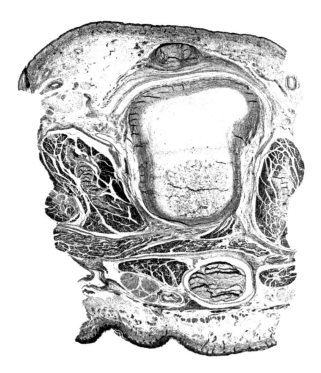

Fig. 5.57 (*series no. 1279*; neg. 21653). Level: 88. Formation of the partition between the second lumbrical and the tendons of the middle finger.

plate in a palmar direction. The distal capsular recess of the meta-carpophalangeal joint becomes visible between the inner anchors (Fig. 5.42), a situation which we will see again in the next section at the end of the analysis of the metacarpophalangeal region.

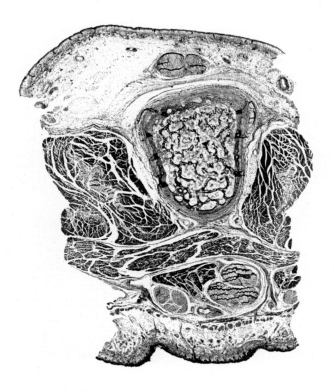

Fig. 5.58 (*series no. 1279*; neg. 21654).
Level: 0. Section through the middle
finger ray, crossed by the proximal palmar
crease and the thenar crease. The partition
walls of the palmar aponeurosis are
formed. Notice the longitudinal fibres in
the wall radial to the second lumbrical.

2. THE METACARPOPHALANGEAL REGION

The analysis is started at a level where the middle ray crosses the
proximal transverse crease of the palm, distinctly proximal to the
metacarpophalangeal joint. The partition walls of the palmar
aponeurosis are just being formed. There is a clear distinction between
the longitudinal strands of the palmar aponeurosis and the transversely arranged layer. We see longitudinal fibres quite clearly in
the partition walls; they are most conspicuous in the wall radial to the
second lumbrical. It is also quite clear that the ulnar aspect of the
compartment is a curved wall, while the radial wall of the still
undivided flexor-lumbrical compartment inclines towards the interosseous fascia forming a sharp niche. In these proximal sections of the
series the adductor pollicis can still be seen in the cross-section. The
extensor tendon is a twin structure situated dorsal to an infratendinous fascial layer. Both the superficial and the deep flexor tendons
are surrounded by a fairly thick peritendineum, separated from the
compartment wall by an areolar layer.

Longitudinal fibres can be seen to penetrate the transverse layer
at more than one place so contributing to the compartment wall
(Fig. 5.58). At this level a synovial cleft has just appeared in the
section, deep to the profundus tendon. At the same levels (Fig. 5.57)
a compartment wall forms between the tendons and the lumbrical-
nerve-vessel area as a protrusion of the deep layer of the palmar
aponeurosis. It seems certain that this protrusion consists of longitudinal fibres. The superficial longitudinal strands of the 'languette'
are somewhat independent of the deep, transversely arranged layer.
The deep longitudinal fibres penetrate the transverse layer from other
directions and at more proximal levels.

The reinforcement of the compartment wall, including its transversely arranged roof, is most striking. We see that the flexor tendons become gradually surrounded by one continuous synovial cleft. The superficial longitudinal strands of the palmar aponeurosis remain visible. Junctions with the skin occur regularly. A most conspicuous feature is the concentration of three, discrete, deep longitudinal bundles, one radial to the lumbrical, one at the junction of the ulnar wall and the adductor fascia and a third in the roof, just between the tendon area and the lumbrical muscle which form the proximal commencement of a septum (Fig. 5.57). The section of Figure 5.56 also shows longitudinal bundles in the compartment walls. The ulnar bundle is just becoming incorporated into the transverse intermetacarpal ligament. The bundle between the lumbrical and the flexor tendons clearly lies in relation to a longitudinal stratum of the palmar aponeurosis, at a level somewhat deeper than the languette of the middle finger which runs free from the underlying layer. This section may well serve as the proximal base for an analysis of the metacarpophalangeal region. At this level both interossei are enclosed in a fascial compartment resulting from a fascial sheet penetrating between each interosseus and the shaft of the metacarpal. The interosseous compartment wall is continuous with the transverse lamina of the extensor assembly. The infratendinous fascia is well marked on the dorsal aspect of the joint and palmarwards becomes a fairly indistinct pericapsular layer. The origin of the metacarpo-glenoidal ligaments lies in or below the infratendineal areolar zone. The areolar space between the interosseous compartment wall and the shaft is traversed by somewhat irregular strands running between the compartment wall and the bone. The related area is fairly rich in vessels and the vascularity continues into the palmar area as strands of vascular tissue lying between the adductor layer and the metacarpal. It is clear that all these features are characteristic of the retroarticular region. The articular cavity opens up and at the same levels conspicuous ligamentous structures become visible. In Figure 5.55 we wish to point out ligaments which originate bilaterally from the head of the metacarpal on the palmar aspect; these ligaments converge on the midline of the metacarpal and are seen largely to reinforce the volar plate of the joint, particularly its juxtametacarpal layer. The same section allows us to mark further contributions to the volar plate. First comes the reinforcement resulting from the formation of the transverse intermetacarpal ligament, then comes the contribution from the interosseous compartment wall, which receives contributions from the transverse lamina and occasionally from an infratendinous layer. At this level the metacarpo-glenoidal ligament, visible on the ulnar aspect as a layer lying lateral to the metacarpophalangeal ligament, starts to become inserted into the volar plate. A fibrous envelope of the tendons is now formed in its entirety and it seems beyond doubt that the ulnar septum and the middle longitudinal bundle are both replaced by either transverse or circular fibres. It is obvious that the transition of a mainly longitudinal structure into a circular structure can hardly be seen to be the result of a continuous transformation. It seems possible, however, that the longitudinal fibres gradually move towards the transverse intermetacarpal ligament and that they are replaced simultaneously by circular fibres, derived from the transverse layer of the palmar aponeurosis. The sheath is firmly anchored into the volar plate bilaterally and reinforces this layer.

While we now see the gradual formation of a rounded ulnar wall of the flexor compartment arising as an extension of the transverse layer of the palmar aponeurosis, we also see that the radial wall extends to the transverse intermetacarpal ligament. This radial wall, however, is mainly composed of longitudinal fibres.

Figure 5.55 is most interesting as it shows (1) the continuity of the transverse aponeurosis layer into the ulnar wall, (2) the formation of the radial wall by longitudinal fibres, (3) a transverse strand above the sheath and (4) longitudinal strands between this layer and the sheath. Above the transverse layer independent longitudinal strands remain visible. It should be noted that the peritendineal layer is still separated from the fibrous sheath by an areolar layer over a considerable part of its circumference. For this reason we might also ask if the term 'compartment wall' is not more proper than 'tendon sheath'. A few sections distally we again see that the longitudinal fibres, deep to the transverse layer of the palmar aponeurosis, also contribute to the compartment wall. There remains a certain independency between the fibrous tendon sheath and the thick volar plate, in so far as an areolar space occurs locally between sheath and ligament layer, without interfering with the strong fibrous anchorages (Fig. 5.54). This areolar space is soon replaced by the joint cavity moving volarwards from two laterally placed capsular pockets. It is obvious that this process involves a displacement of the ligaments reinforcing the volar plate. A retroarticular fibrous bridge has existed so far, between the volar plate and laterally placed ligaments. The expansion of the joint cavity enables the laterally originating ligaments to reinforce the fibrous floor of the tendon sheath so that it now becomes a massive volar plate. We should also note that (Fig. 5.54) a metacarpo-glenoidal ligament represents a layer lying lateral to the metacarpophalangeal bundle, as well as a ligament lying in palmar continuity with the metacarpophalangeal bundle. On the radial aspect a strong inner interosseous compartment wall is fused with the metacarpo-glenoidal bundle and is most conspicuous. The ligaments from the palmar side of the metacarpal head remain in the juxtacapsular part of the plate. The structure of the volar plate will be observed later in a sagittal series.

In later sections pertaining to the metacarpal head, the volar plate and the transverse intermetacarpal ligament, we see the following developments: (1) a gradual insertion of the superficial longitudinal palmar aponeurosis strands into the skin, (2) the emergence of the webspace, (3) the division of the volar digital nerve and (4) the division of the second interosseous compartment by an extension of the transverse lamina.

An interruption in the transverse layer of the palmar aponeurosis is a regular feature and the emergence of a new transverse strand again takes place so that longitudinal strands become located deep to the transverse layer (Fig. 5.53). These longitudinal strands merge into the flexor tendon envelope. The envelope now inclines on both sides towards the transverse intermetacarpal ligament. The joint cavity extends around the metacarpal capitulum, as far as the origin of the metacarpophalangeal ligaments. The layer lateral to these

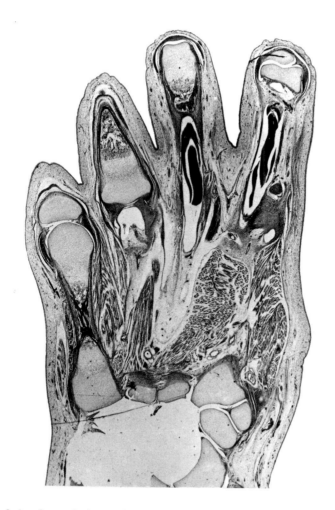

Fig. 6.14 (*series no. 1280*; neg. 24245).
This section provides information on the
inter-relationships between the palmar
aponeurosis compartment, the tendon
sheath of metacarpophalangeal level and
the tendon sheath of phalanx I. Palmar IV
forms the radial wing in the little finger.

border of the first phalanx sheath segment in this finger. The next
figure (6.12) is an enlargement and shows in detail the ulnar side
of the fourth finger; we can see that the wing tendon complex
passes in front of the transverse lamina and its major part continues
into the wing. An inner tendon fascicle is seen to join the
phalangeal insertion of this same muscle. In Figure 6.13 the tendon
sheath of the medius has also been opened. We see a marked border
between the sheath of the first phalanx and the metacarpophalangeal
segment of the sheath derived from the volar plate. This border for the
index finger is equally apparent in this figure. A conspicuous vascular
hilum is visible at this spot.

We now see a number of interesting features. Figure 6.14 shows
that the metacarpophalangeal sheath of the medius ends distally in
one or two spurs, identical with the distal extensions from the volar
plate at more dorsal levels. Hence the inner spur is layer-wise
identical with the outer anchor of the volar plate, or with the suspensory system of the metacarpophalangeal tendon sheath which is
virtually the same system. It seems quite important to stress the fact
that the tendon sheath volar plate system extends distally into a
radiating system that diverges into the skin, while its inner components
converge upon the phalangeal base. At more palmar levels it is essential
to examine the proximal continuities of the tendon sheaths.

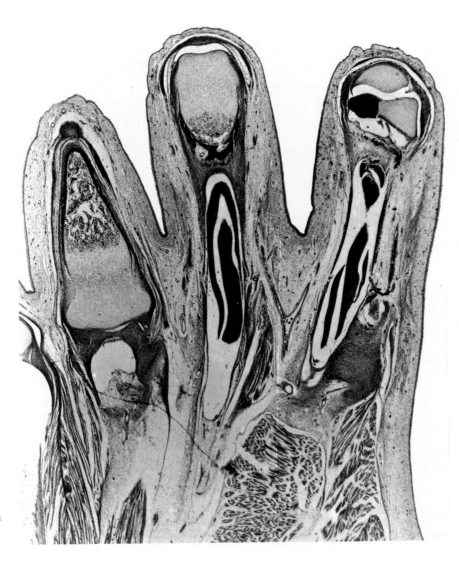

Fig. 6.15 (*series no. 1280*; neg. 24252).
Frontal section through the tendon sheath
and the tendon compartments of the
index and medius.

In Figure 6.15 we are faced with a remarkable situation. First we
notice the pronounced gap between the segment of the metacarpophalangeal sheath and the segment of the first phalanx and it is
obvious that this is a site of vascular entrance. Secondly, we notice
that the proximal continuation of the metacarpophalangeal segment
of the sheath divides proximally into a synovial layer and a fibrous
layer which is obviously the compartment wall of the palmar
aponeurosis. In other words there exists here a marked areolar
space between the synovial sheath and the compartment wall, a
space that does not exist between the sheath present at metacarpophalangeal level and its synovial layer.

While the compartment wall and metacarpophalangeal sheath are
in close contact with each other, very careful observation shows a
distinct difference in texture within the structures involved, at many
places. There is no interruption of fibrous tissue by, e.g. a cleft, but
the separateness of the two layers is made quite distinct by the pattern
of the texture.

Figure 6.16 is very informative about the relationship of the

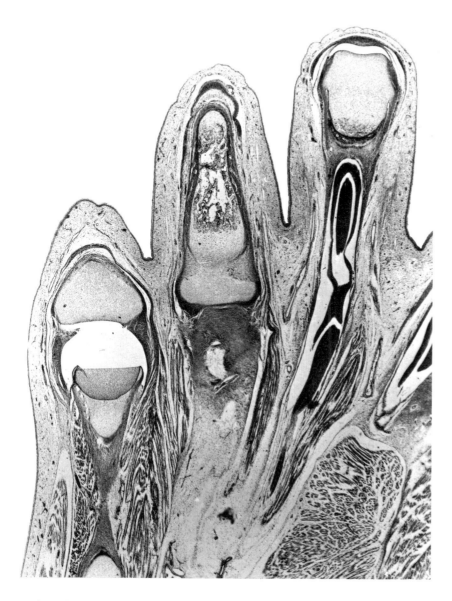

Fig. 6.16 (*series no. 1280*; neg. 24254). The proximo-distal composition of the tendon sheath of the medius, commencing proximally with the palmar aponeurosis compartment.

tendon sheath compartment wall to the middle finger. Compartment wall and synovial sheath are, as usual, separated from each other by an areolar space and the synovial sheath is directly transformed into the fibrous tendon sheath at metacarpophalangeal level, again the usual situation. On both sides the compartment wall and synovial sheath come increasingly close together until they appear to be continuous with each other. We believe, however, that the situation enables us to distinguish a free proximal border of the fibrous sheath. There are fibrous extensions from the compartment wall passing distally and the tendon sheath shows thin layers developing from it which pass distally. Figure 6.16 is also a good picture of the formation of the wing by palmar IV on the radial side of the little finger.

Further information regarding the relationship between compartment wall and tendon sheath (and subsequently between various tendon sheath segments) is found in a figure such as 6.17. In the middle finger we see a compartment wall neatly derived from the

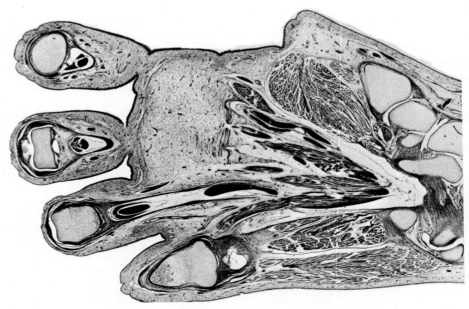

Fig. 6.18 (*series no. 1280*; neg. 15038). The natatorial system, the transverse system of the palmar aponeurosis and the transitions in the tendon sheath of the ring finger.

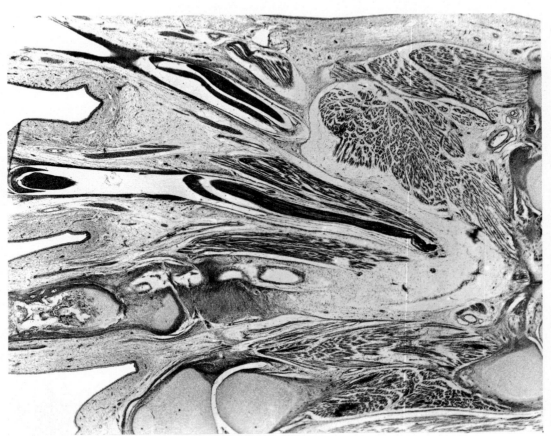

Fig. 6.17 (*series no. 1280*; neg. 24253). The transition of the palmar aponeurosis tendon compartment into the metacarpophalangeal sheath section in the index and medius.

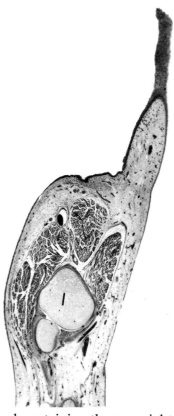

Fig. 6.19 (*series no. 2118*; neg. 21147). Section brushing the radial side of the index. I = metacarpal I.

palmar aponeurosis and containing the synovial tendon sheath separated by an areolar space. Distally the latter sheath becomes the fibrous tendon sheath at metacarpophalangeal level. The palmar aponeurosis ends by forming spurs in the surrounding tissue. From the metacarpophalangeal segment of the tendon sheath fascial layers are seen to pass into the surrounding tissues. The innermost layer passes into the tendon sheath at the level of the first phalanx. In passing we see that we have opened up the sheath of the volar nerve-vessel bundle.

Figure 6.18 shows a slightly different situation regarding the tendon sheath of the ring finger. The sheath segments at meta-carpophalangeal and at phalanx I levels are continuous and can be distinguished from each other by virtue of their respective internal patterns: the metacarpophalangeal segment has a tapering shape and while the greater part of the first phalanx segment is uniformly thick, its distal end increases in thickness. The metacarpophalangeal segment is seen to give off a thin layer into the surrounding tissue. The compartment wall on the radial side is entirely independent from the synovial sheath and does not extend into the sheath proper at metacarpophalangeal levels.

Finally this last section permits us to make some interesting obser-vations on the natatorial system and on the transverse components of the palmar aponeurosis.

SERIES No. 2118

We have examined a sagittally cut series in order to check the findings

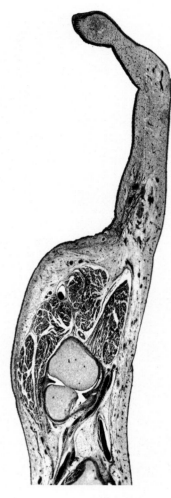

Fig. 6.20 (*series no. 2118*; neg. 21148).
This is a section of the proximal root of
the digital band.

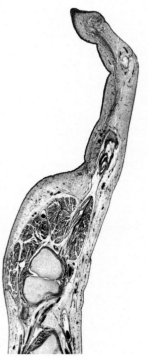

Fig. 6.21 (*series no. 2118*; neg. 21149).
The distal extension of the digital band.
Notice the layers of the
metacarpophalangeal joint, including the
extensor hood.

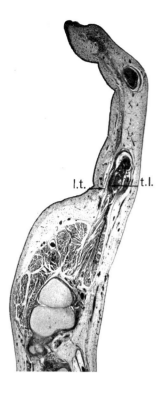

Fig. 6.22 (*series no. 2118*; neg. 21150). A tangential section of the metacarpophalangeal joint and the proximal interphalangeal joint. l.t. = lumbrical tendon; t.l. = transverse lamina.

gathered in the transverse series so far and to extend our observations to those relationships which are poorly seen in transverse sections. This series will be described in a radioulnar sequence.

The section seen in Figure 6.19 comes very close to the radial side of the index and the extension of the palmar aponeurosis into the subcorial layer of the thenar is visible. In the next figure (6.20) we see the marked fibrous anchor originating from the subcorial area in the thenar region. This anchor is located external to the radial nerve-vessel bundle of the index. The connection of this system to the superficial layers of the joint region, viz. the transverse lamina and its delaminations, is clearly seen in Figure 6.21 which is immediately adjacent to the fibrous structures of the metacarpophalangeal joint. The extensor assembly is seen receiving the lumbrical tendon and a tiny extension from the transverse lamina near the volar plate. In this figure the digital band is cut along its entire length.

The first dorsal interosseus has appeared in the section of Figure 6.22. Some bundles of this muscle are inserted into the transverse lamina on its palmar aspect. In this figure we see a fibrous layer below the transverse lamina and this is obviously the infratendineal layer blending with the periosteum at the base of the phalanx. The width of the first interosseous tendon is quite striking and it is clear that its major insertion is into the phalangeal base. The section of the proximal interphalangeal joint shows the extensor assembly lying as a cap over the joint area proper. We can see quite clearly the continuity of the distal portion of the so-called digital band with an outer periligamentous layer and although the structure of the ligament layer is somewhat diffuse, the main fibre trend is from a dorso-proximal origin to a distovolar insertion. In this same section we can trace a thin fibrous continuity between the lumbrical fascia and the skin anchoring system and see that, in its turn, the lumbrical fascia is

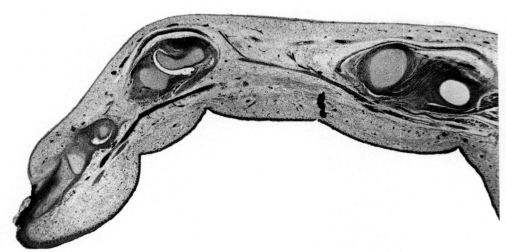

Fig. 6.24 (*series no. 2118*; neg. 21151). The dorsal branch of the volar digital nerve is seen cut along its whole length. The section gives a good view of the radial metacarpophalangeal ligament.

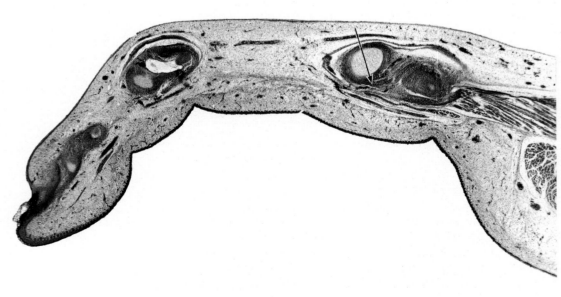

Fig. 6.23 (*series no. 2118*; neg. 21164). The three joints of the chain seen in this picture are largely tangential in section. The insertion of the metacarpophalangeal bundle is indicated by an arrow. Both the lumbrical and the volar nerve have appeared in this section.

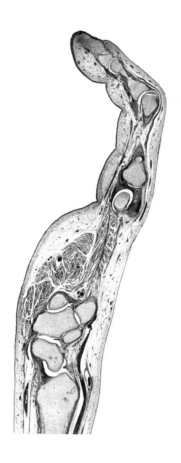

Fig. 6.25 (*series no. 2118*; neg. 21152). The three joints of the finger are seen just medial to their ligament walls. Notice the volar plates of the joints and their anchorages.

continuous with the palmar interosseous fascia. In the next section (Fig. 6.23) we see that both the lumbrical and the nerve compartments are open. This section and the next give a good picture of the extensor hood, of the infratendineal fascia blending with the periosteum of the first phalanx, and the conspicuous oblique course of the radial metacarpophalangeal ligament. It is noticeable that the interosseous tendon and the transverse lamina can barely be distinguished from each other. The ligaments of the distal interphalangeal joint can also be seen in this section and although they have a felt-like appearance, it is beyond doubt that the main direction of the fibres is from dorsoproximal to distovolar.

Figure 6.24 shows a most instructive section. The dorsoradial branch of the volar nerve is cut along a considerable portion of its length. It runs lateral to the radial volar digital artery. The lumbrical muscle and tendon are seen and the extensor assembly has a free lateral border, though enveloped in a fascial structure which blends with volar capsular structures. The distinct oblique course of the metacarpophalangeal ligament is very clearly seen. The conjoint transverse lamina and interosseous tendon fascicles are still separated from the metacarpoglenoidal ligaments by an areolar cleft. These ligaments originate from the metacarpal head and could be seen in previous sections. It becomes clear in subsequent sections that various layers fuse into the volar plate of the joint. In both this section and the previous one the attachment of the volar plate of

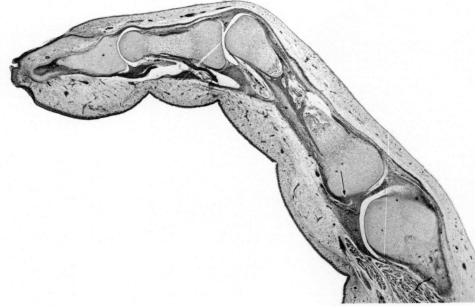

Fig. 6.27 (*series no. 2118*; neg. 21166). The radial sublimis fascicle is seen being inserted into the middle phalanx. Note the arch over the vascular area of the proximal interphalangeal joint. In the metacarpophalangeal joint we just see the metacarpophalangeal ligament (arrow) and above it the inner distal anchor of the volar plate.

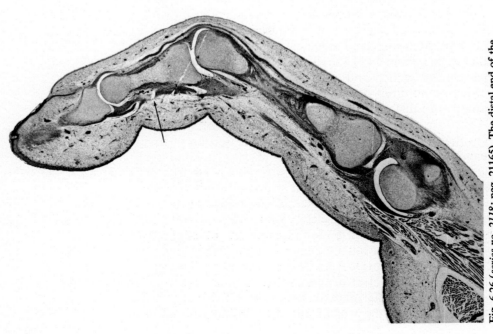

Fig. 6.26 (*series no. 2118*; neg. 21165). The distal end of the tendon sheath is opened. Note the continuity of the distal tendon sheath segment into the tendon sheath section of phalanx II (arrow).

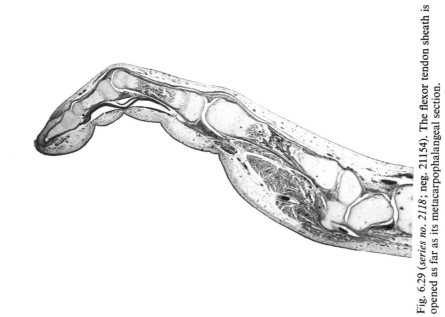

Fig. 6.29 (*series no. 2118*; neg. 21154). The flexor tendon sheath is opened as far as its metacarpophalangeal section.

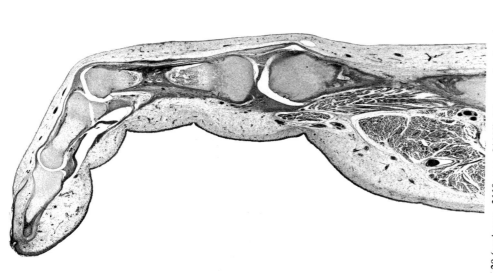

Fig. 6.28 (*series no. 2118*; neg. 21153). The proximal anchor of the proximal interphalangeal section of the tendon sheath is clearly visible.

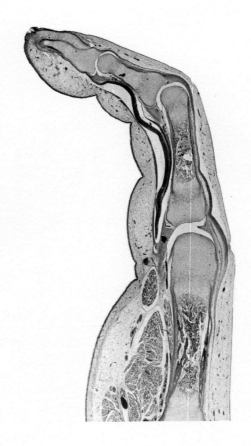

Fig. 6.30 (*series no. 2118*; neg. 21155).
The tendon sheath has been opened from
its distal tip as far as the
metacarpophalangeal region. Note the
vascular bed of profundus and sublimis
proximal to the proximal interphalangeal
joint.

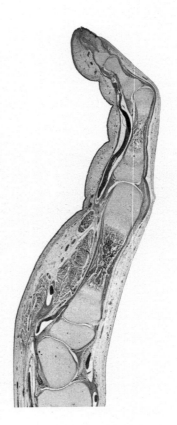

Fig. 6.31 (*series no. 2118*; neg. 21156).
Section showing the palmar aponeurosis
derived compartment wall, the synovial
sheath contained within the compartment
and the sections of the tendon sheath
proper.

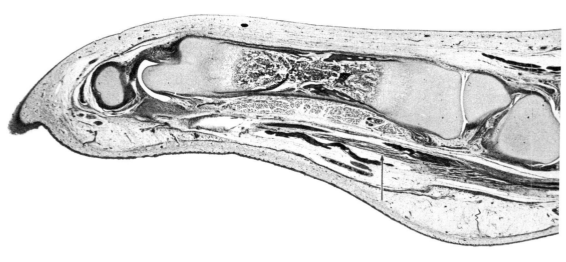

Fig. 6.45 (*series no. 2118*; neg. 24394). Tangential section through the radial side of the medius. We see here a deep palmar aponeurosis radiation into the fibrous constellation of the metacarpophalangeal region. Notice the fascial duplicature enclosing the wing of the assembly and a fascial delamination of the wing lying over it. arrow=lumbrical II.

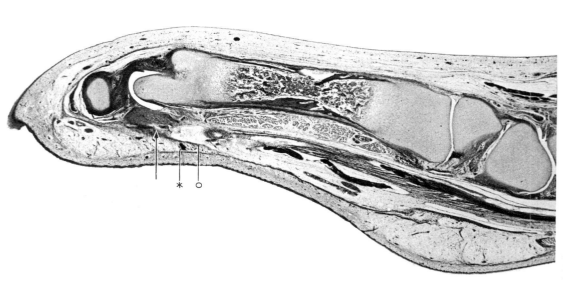

Fig. 6.44 (*series no. 2118*; neg. 24393). Superficial (*) and deep palmar aponeurosis (○) strands extending into the subcorial layer of the webspace and into pericapsular metacarpophalangeal layers. Notice the transverse fibres of the palmar aponeurosis lying just between the two strands. The arrow indicates the septum on the radial side of the long finger flexors.

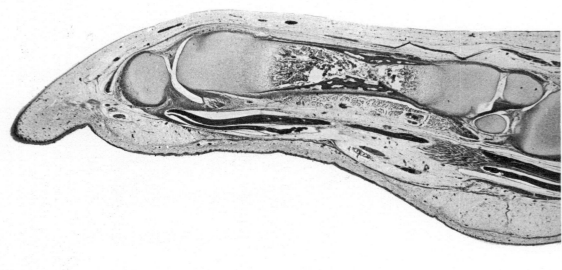

Fig. 6.47 (*series no. 2118; neg. 24396*). The metacarpophalangeal sheath section in tangential section. Notice the palmar aponeurosis derived compartment wall which extends distally as a thin fascia over the metacarpophalangeal sheath.

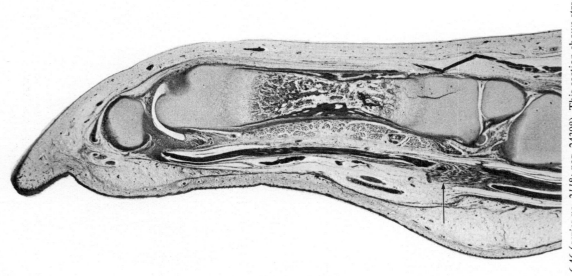

Fig. 6.46 (*series no. 2118; neg. 24398*). This section shows strands of the palmar aponeurosis continuing into subcorial layers of the webspace, while more dorsally directed strands constitute the compartment surrounding the synovial tendon sheath. The compartment wall continues distally over the metacarpophalangeal sheath as a fascial layer. arrow = lumbrical III.

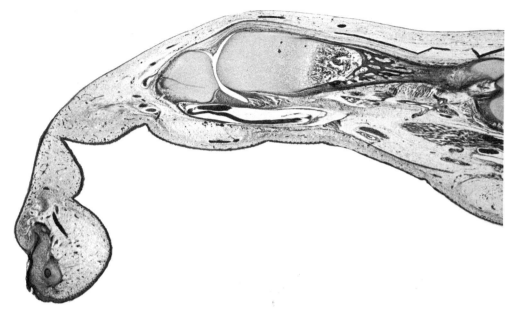

Fig. 6.49 (*series no. 2118*; neg. 24401). Section showing the nerve-vessel sheath at the base of the finger and its position with respect to the natatorial ligament and the digital band. Notice the two layers in the volar capsule of the metacarpophalangeal joint, a juxtametacarpal layer and a volar plate proper.

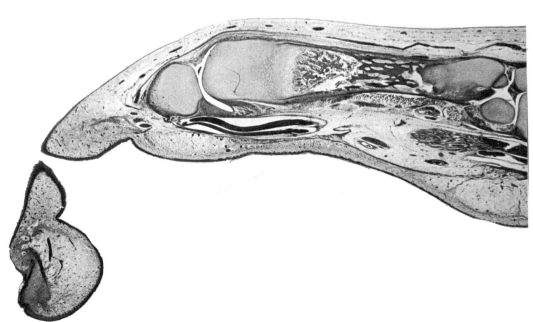

Fig. 6.48 (*series no. 2118*; neg. 24397). Except for the relations pictured in Fig. 6.47 this figure shows the digital band related to the natatorial ligament. A nerve branch passes dorsally (cf. Fig. 6.49). The two layers in the volar capsule of the metacarpophalangeal joint are extremely conspicuous.

such as 6.37 and 6.38 the layer of the transverse fibres is seen to be involved in septum formation by means of vertical strands which seem to be derived from this layer (Fig. 6.39).

We should now try to integrate some of the observations made in the transverse series with those made in the sagittal sections. One general feature dominates the scene of transformation between midhand and finger and that is the continuity of fascial and fibrous structures. There is much evidence for the continuity of the longitudinal palmar aponeurosis system into the compartments and continuities of the latter into fascial hoods around tendon sheaths at metacarpophalangeal level, although very thin, are unmistakable (Fig. 6.35). Figures 6.37 and 6.38 also provide evidence for the proximal origin of the digital band from the site of fusion between a septum and the transverse intermetacarpal ligament.

Sections through the webspace (Figs. 6.40 to 6.46) are most informative on continuities of the transverse intermetacarpal ligament that join the extensor assembly as a fascial layer. It is distinctive in Figure 6.42 that this fascial layer, delaminated from the extensor assembly, can be traced in a proximal direction palmar of the lumbrical as far as the subcorial extension of the palmar aponeurosis. Another feature is the fibrofascial spur derived from the natatorial ligament which passes dorsally. The fibres become lost in the supratendineal or subcutaneous fascial layer. In these sections the free border of the wing of the extensor assembly is held in a fascial duplicature as in the transverse series. In the transverse series this fascial duplicature was a derivative of the suspensory system of the volar plate and tendon sheath. In the present series we can only be sure that this layer is derived from the volar plate. In Figure 6.45 the continuity visible between the palmar aponeurosis, a compartment wall and this fascial layer, is not at variance with the afore-mentioned continuity. The only point is that transverse series permit a more precise discrimination of various components of the capsular fibrous system. When we consider continuities into the digital band it seems appropriate to refer to the observations made in the horizontal series. We recall that the distal radiations from the volar plates, comprising both the outer anchors of these plates, passed into the phalangeal bases as well as the digital bands and that the latter coursed dorsal to the nerve-vessel bundle.

A point now to be tackled concerns the fate of the longitudinal strands of the aponeurosis that run as the so-called 'languettes' superficial to the transverse system. Because these superficial fibres are arranged like the rays of the hand, it is not surprising that they are absent from some sections. A good example of a languette extending into subcorial layers in the roof of the webspace just over the joint can be found in Figure 6.42.

Figure 6.46 reveals the layer-wise position (1) of the compartment wall derived from the palmar aponeurosis and extending into a fascial hood over the metacarpophalangeal part of the sheath, (2) of the natatorial ligament, (3) of the inner and outer leaves of the nerve-vessel envelope, (4) of the digital band in the dorsal margin of this envelope and finally (5) of the fascial envelope of the wing.

A few sections will be added just to check some of the points raised in the course of this survey. Figure 6.47 shows the radial side

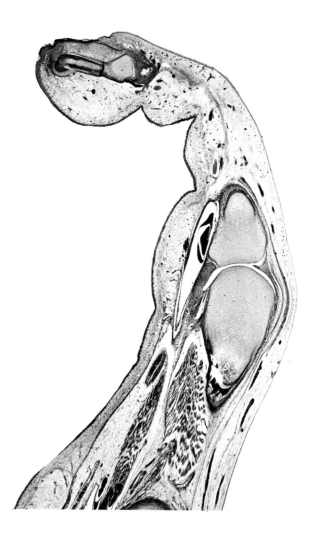

Fig. 6.50 (*series no. 2118*; neg. 24402). Tangential section of the radial side of the medius. This section gives some evidence of both longitudinal and transverse components of the palmar aponeurosis contributing to the formation of a septum, or compartment wall.

of the medius and provides a clear example of the participation of a deep longitudinal palmar aponeurosis strand in the formation of a compartment wall, and of the layer-wise position of the metacarpophalangeal sheath. The latter is continuous with the synovial layer within the compartment, whereas the compartment wall seems to lose itself just above the sheath.

Figure 6.48 shows the radiation of the digital band into the finger next to the natatorial ligament in cross-section. Figure 6.49 is of interest as it shows the dorsal passage of the dorsal branch of the volar digital nerve and the contribution of the natatorial ligament to the formation of the digital band. In this respect it is perhaps useful to emphasize that the distal extension of the natatorial ligament itself is located more on the volar side than in the digital band. Figure 6.50 gives a good view of the location of these two systems. In Figure 6.51 dorsal branches of the volar digital nerve are found on the radial side of the medius. The proximal branch is the extension of the dorsal branch seen in Figure 6.49. It is obvious that a second branch passes dorsal to the distal interphalangeal joint on its proximal aspect. Figure 6.52 shows conclusively the existence of a proximal anchor of the volar plate of the proximal interphalangeal joint. This

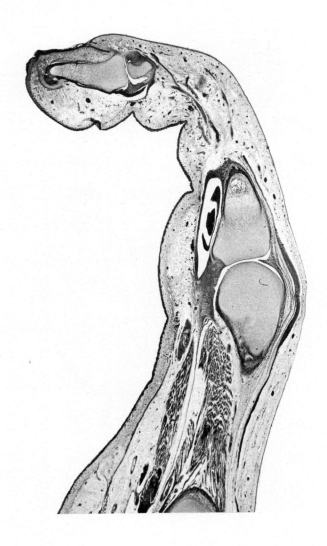

Fig. 6.51 (*series no. 2118*; neg. 24403).
Dorsal branches of the volar digital nerve
passing over the first and second phalanges.
Radial side; medius.

anchor is placed fairly laterally in the finger. The natatorial ligament
just touches the fascial hood over the sheath of the first phalanx.
Figure 6.53 is a sagittal section of the tendon sheath showing the
segment of the second phalanx, the proximal interphalangeal segment
and the segment of the first phalanx; all three of them are seen as
separate units.

Figure 6.54 is a good view of the proximal anchor of the volar
plate of the proximal interphalangeal joint on the ulnar side of the
medius. Both the natatorial system and the digital band can be seen,
the latter being continuous with delaminations from the extensor
hood. We found minute dorsal branches from the volar digital nerve
on this side of the finger passing along the first and third phalanges.
On the radial side of the ring finger a very conspicuous proximal
anchor of the volar plate can be seen. Figure 6.56 shows a view of
this same anchor on the ulnar side of this finger. On this side we
failed to trace a marked dorsal nerve branch, although minute dorsal
branches could be present. Analysis in this series would not be
feasible for the little finger because the section was semi-frontal and
semi-sagittal.

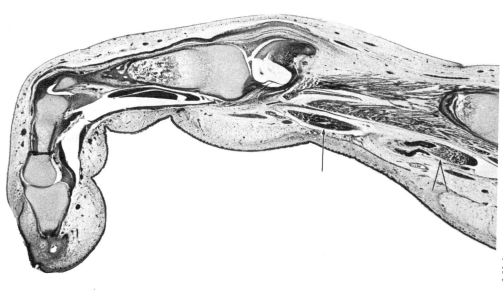

Fig. 6.53 (*series no. 2118*; neg. 24405). Section passing through the tendon sheath of the middle finger. arrow = lumbrical III; double-stemmed arrow = lumbrical IV.

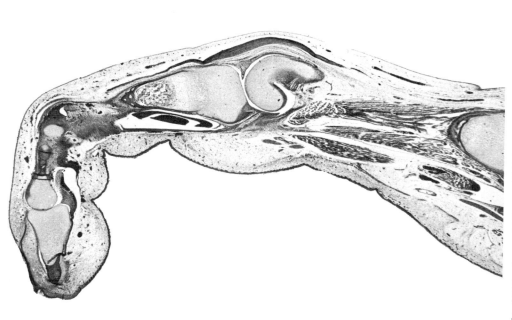

Fig. 6.52 (*series no. 2118*; neg. 24404). Sagittal section through the radial side of the middle finger.

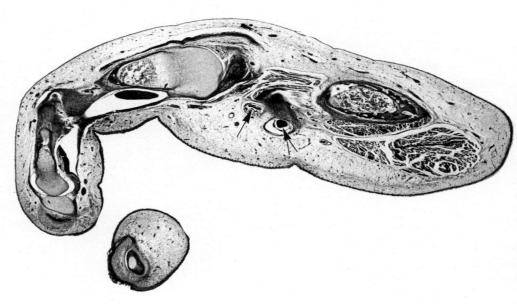

Fig. 6.55 (*series no. 2118*; neg. 24407). Section through the radial side of the phalanges of the ring finger. arrow=lumbrical IV; double-stemmed arrow=flexor tendon of the fifth metacarpal.

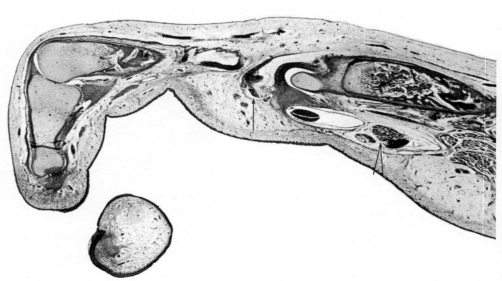

Fig. 6.54 (*series no. 2118*; neg. 24406). Section through the ulnar side of the medius and through the radial side of the fourth metacarpal. arrow=lumbrical III; double-stemmed arrow=lumbrical IV.

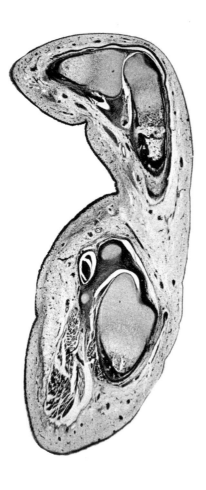

Fig. 6.56 (*series no. 2118*; neg. 24408). Section through the ulnar side of the ring finger and through the metacarpophalangeal joint of the little finger.

7. Microdissection

In order to check the validity of the cross-section analysis and the applicability of its results we carried out microdissections of the hand. It is not surprising that, unlike a dissection based on systemic principles, the exploration of the hand can be endlessly varied. For this reason we chose the routes that most satisfied the requirements of producing maximum information and of being easily reproducible.

1. THE ULNAR APPROACH

Exploration of the Subcutaneous Hypothenar Area

1. The first dissection was carried out on a left hand (adult) (Figs. 7.1 and 7.2).

The skin was incised longitudinally along the palmar aspect of the hypothenar area and reflected on both sides for a short distance only. From this incision the exploration was carried out as far as possible by blunt dissection. Our microscopic findings directed this dissection towards some specific points.

First, the fibrous skin anchors, derived from the pisiform bone, were preserved. Secondly, we tried to locate the palmaris brevis layer, dissecting bluntly through the fatty layer and also the floor of the hypothenar area distal to the palmaris brevis. From this level, blunt dissection continued medially, i.e. along the inner border of the hypothenar area. Immediately proximal to the palmaris brevis the exploration of the fatty tissue leads easily to the ulnar nerve and vessels on the inner side of the pisiform bone lying on the flexor retinaculum. From this area a typical fatty pad can be removed, partly from below the palmaris brevis; the same pad was seen microscopically in our sections.

The hamulus ossis hamati can be located and also the pisiform-hamulus ligament (lig. pisohamatum). The deep branches of the ulnar nerve and vessels can be exposed where they separate from the superficial branches.

The palmaris brevis is extremely well developed in this preparation. The ulnar insertion into, or its origin from, the skin, can be established. The individual muscular fascicles give rise to a tendon plate, in which fibrous strands can be traced in various directions. Openings between fascicles reflect the fascicle-type structure of the plate. Preparing this layer medially, one approaches the skin and there is an impression received that the muscle is inserted into the skin; this is not the case, however, although at the inner border of the hypothenar area fibrous skin insertions from various sources do occur, as we will see presently.

The dissection beyond the palmaris brevis medially leads to the ulnar wall of the flexor compartment and is arrested there. We cannot reach the midhand subcutaneous area, at least not very deeply, because of the anchorage of the flexor compartment wall to the skin. Beyond the distal transverse crease, dissection denudes the flexor sheath of the little finger and leads easily into the webspace between the fourth and fifth fingers.

The result of the exploration is presented in Figure 7.1. The drawing serves as a guide for orientation and for the findings which

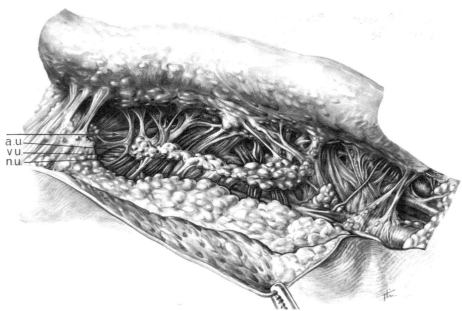

a.u.
v.u.
n.u.

Fig. 7.1 (T. 1266; neg. 18730). An exploration of the subcutaneous hypothenar space
The palmaris brevis, the deep ulnar root of the palmar aponeurosis, the skin anchorage
of the latter and the dense fibrous strands anchoring the skin to the ulnar wall of the
flexor tendon compartment have been exposed. Notice also the offshoots of the palmaris
brevis into the longitudinal system. Various small vascular and nervous branches have
been exposed. The arrow indicates the ulnar root of the palmar aponeurosis. a.u. =
a.ulnaris; v.u. = v.ulnaris; n.u. = n.ulnaris.

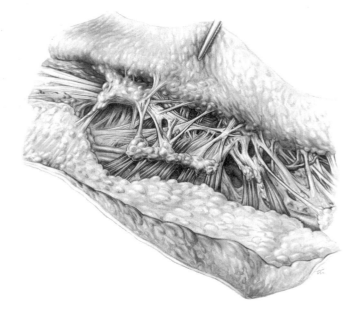

Fig. 7.2 (T. 1503; 23253). An exploration
of the subcutaneous hypothenar space.
The palmaris brevis, the deep ulnar root of
the palmar aponeurosis, the skin anchorage
of the latter and the dense fibrous strands
anchoring the skin to the ulnar wall of the
flexor tendon compartment have been
exposed. Notice also the offshoots of
the palmaris brevis into the longitudinal
system. Various small vascular and nervous
branches have been exposed.

will be presented now. The skin anchor of the pisiform bone runs
mediodistally towards the skin. The ulnar nerve and vessels are easily
seen. Exploration of the flexor retinaculum brings the longitudinal
bundle into view and this can be traced proximally below the ulnar
nerve and vessels into the pisiform area or its distal extension, the
pisohamate ligament. The relation of the longitudinal bundle to the
flexor retinaculum is very intimate; it cannot be isolated fully from

more transversely running fibres, but it can be followed as a bundle
with a free lateral border, running over the palmaris brevis and
towards its skin anchorage halfway along the inner border of the
hypothenar eminence. In the drawing this skin anchor is hidden from
view by fatty tissue. It can also be seen that this lateral border is
rounded by fascial strands derived from the palmaris brevis all along
its length; these strands often contain some vascular branches and
it is also evident that more tendinous fascicles derived from the
palmaris brevis either join the lateral free border, or else pass along
it to become inserted into the skin. One of the palmaris brevis strands
is seen to pass in a proximomedial direction (it is the second strand
in the drawing) as it joins subcorial strata. The branched structure
that follows contains some small vessels and then we see a bundle
extending along the lateral border and also forming an attachment
to the skin. Distal to this bundle in the same drawing, there are quite
a few palmaris brevis fibres which pass into the main skin anchorage.

On further exploration (Fig. 7.2) we found the longitudinal bundle
lying deep in the preparation and it was found that this bundle joins
the palmar aponeurosis plate to form its lateral border as far as
'midway' skin anchorage: hence the bundle represents the deep ulnar
root of the palmar aponeurosis. Access to the palmar surface of the
aponeurosis is considerably hampered, not only by the skin anchors
described but also by deeper skin attachments which pass between
the longitudinal fascicles of the palmar aponeurosis.

We now return to the point where palmaris brevis fibres joined the
longitudinal strand and were found to be inserted into the skin, an
anchorage obscured in the first drawing (Fig. 7.1) by the fatty pad.
In this area we see the proximal origin of strands from the skin which
join the inner hypothenar wall distally.

In both drawings we see that the distal palmaris brevis fascicles
are oriented in a more or less laterodistal medioproximal direction.

We now touch upon the system that contributes to the formation
of the ulnar wall of the flexor tendon compartment and that closes
off the midpalmar subcutaneous space at its border with the subcutaneous hypothenar area. This fairly dense pillar-system consists
of strong sloping fibres which run distally towards the hypothenar
fascia. By making a small hole in the hypothenar fascia we could see
the proximal border of the ulnar flexor compartment wall.

2. The second dissection was carried out also on a left hand (Figs.
7.3, 7.4 and 7.5).

The results of this dissection are also shown in a number of
drawings. The first drawing (Fig. 7.3) is a fairly rough sketch intended
as a general view of the situation present after the first stage of our
dissection. The dorsal branch of the ulnar nerve is prepared, one
branch passes to the ulnodorsal side of the little finger, the other is
the nerve prior to its branching for the adjacent sides of the little
and ring fingers and for the radial side of the latter. The nerve has
rounded the styloid process of the ulna and is running over the
reinforced fascia of the hypothenar compartment. Just above it we
see the terminal track of the flexor carpi ulnaris near its insertion into
the pisiform bone.

From our microscopical findings it is not surprising that the

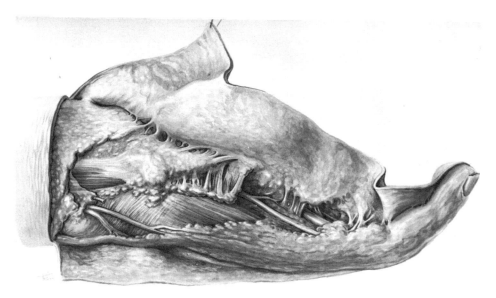

Fig. 7.3 (T. 891; neg. 13297). Drawing of the situation after the first stage of an exploration of the subcutaneous hypothenar space. The dorsal ulnar nerve has been dissected, which makes it possible to locate the styloid process of the ulna. The flexor carpi ulnaris leads to the pisiform area, from which strong anchors radiate into the skin. The palmaris brevis is also attached to the skin. The ulnovolar nerve of the little finger is seen distal to this structure. The tendon sheath of the fifth finger appears through a fibrous arch.

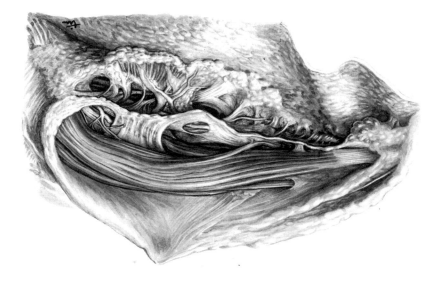

Fig. 7.4 (T. 1236; neg. 18082). Dissection of the hypothenar muscular area and of the overlying subcutaneous area. The 'midway' skin anchor and some of its proximal anchors are exposed. Note the radiation from this anchor into the depth of the preparation.

dissection of the skin entails the division of numerous tiny fibrous connections between it and the fascia of the hypothenar compartment. However, extremely strong anchors to the skin arise from the pisiform in both transverse and more longitudinal directions. The anchors have been left untouched. They are quite visible in the drawing. When the palmaris brevis is exposed again we find that the medial exploration is impeded by numerous connections between the skin and this layer; these are extremely dense at the musculotendinous junction. Because we wished to dissect below this muscle we had to prepare free its ulnar insertion; the result is shown in Figure 7.3.

Fig. 7.5 (T. 1420; neg. 21097). A drawing made of a preparation in a stage of dissection following that in Fig. 7.4. The palmaris brevis is reflected towards the skin so that the longitudinal system, its origin, its skin anchorage and its continuity into the ulnar compartment wall are all accessible. Ramifications of the ulnar digital nerve are shown. The most ulnar longitudinal strand of the palmar aponeurosis is just visible as it is inserted into the skin. The webspace between the fourth and the fifth can be approached over the flexor tunnel of the fifth finger. * = the superficial opponens layer; ○ = muscle belly from the opponens compartment passing to the phalangeal base; arrow = bundles from the abductor proper to ○; black dots: see text.

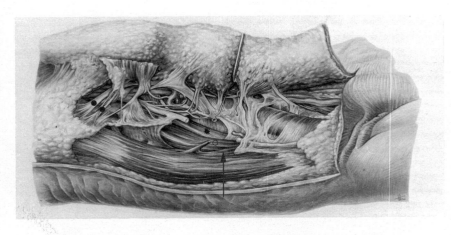

The junction of the palmaris brevis to the skin has been left untouched. Below the palmaris brevis the branch of the volar ulnar nerve to the little finger has been exposed in the hypothenar fascia. Towards the midpalmar area the route is blocked by fairly dense fibrous anchors between the ulnar wall of the hypothenar compartment and the skin, but distal to the distal crease of the palm it is easier to pass over the flexor tunnel towards the webspace between the fifth and fourth fingers. The flexor tendon enclosed in its sheath appears through a form of fibrous arch, which is the distal exit from the compartment of the palmar aponeurosis. Finally this drawing shows strong and dense skin anchorages at the level of the basal digital crease and at the proximal interphalangeal crease.

We continued the exploration and because our cross-section findings have convinced us of the importance of skin anchorages on the inner side of the hypothenar eminence, we decided to pass below the palmaris brevis. It is obvious that this route leads towards the flexor retinaculum and to the space below the palmar aponeurosis, although the route is far from being a free passage. It turns out that fibrous strands arise from both the pisiform and the abductor, or more generally from the hypothenar fascia; strands which become involved in the palmaris brevis layer and which can be traced through this layer into a most conspicuous skin anchorage.

Let us examine this system closely as shown in Figure 7.4 after the second dissection. This drawing was made after a dissection of the muscular area and it therefore serves a double purpose; but in this chapter we will confine ourselves mainly to the subcutaneous region of the drawing. It should be noticed that proximal to the palmaris brevis and below the pisiform skin anchor of Figure 7.3, exploration leads easily to the ulnar nerve-vessel bundle. The approach requires the removal of a fatty body that was already observed by Kirk (1924) and by Frohse (1906) and is readily visible in a section such as Figure 1.4.

As we open the muscular area we find the deep branch of the ulnar nerve with the arterial branch for the muscular space and further exploration concerns the area proximal to the origin of the opponens and the flexor digiti minimi. The lateral surface of the hamulus can be brought into view, as well as the fascicle of the pisometacarpal ligament that skirts the hamulus towards its insertion into the fourth metacarpal; they could not be shown, however, in this drawing. Exploration below the palmaris brevis leads to the isolation of the fibrous system mentioned and also to tiny nerve and arterial branches which reach the subcutaneous areas through the palmaris brevis.

One fibrous anchor from the pisiform area and two more strands from the abductor fascia are seen in Figure 7.4. They fuse with each other as they run below the palmaris brevis and they direct our eye to the strong skin anchorage just halfway along the inner border of the hypothenar eminence, although their continuity into this anchor is hidden by a pad of fat not removed at this stage of the dissection. The situation is far more complicated than could be inferred from this brief description and in order to explain this situation it is necessary to give a detailed report of various structures and to refer repeatedly to the drawings. It will be helpful to include a further stage of dissection in this analysis (Fig. 7.5).

The most proximal pisiform anchor and the first anchor from the abductor fascia (black dots in Fig. 7.5) together form a flat layer of fibres that fans out below the palmaris brevis and blends medially with this layer; laterally the border continues distalwards, also lying below the palmaris brevis as we found previously. Notice that a small artery passes between the two fascicles of this fan and another small branch of this same artery skirts its distal border. This pisiform anchor passes over the superficial branches of the ulnar nerve-vessel bundle. The tip of the hamulus can be seen below this bundle and from the tip a fascial fold is seen joining the abductor fascia. This fold separates the deep and superficial branches of the ulnar nerve and vessels from each other and is the proximal border of the superficial opponens compartment.

The second anchor has a broad fan-like origin from the abductor fascia. The proximal border of this fan is a tiny but strong strand that continues directly into the skin anchorage, which again is skirted distally by a small nerve, a branch from the ulno-volar nerve of the little finger, which divides into two on each side of a small artery, heading for the skin. It is now necessary to comment further on the arrangement of this skin anchor and its relation to other structures in the hand.

As we have seen, the anchors act as a deep fibrous reinforcement of the palmaris brevis and distally the system acts as a deep reinforcement of the palmar aponeurosis. On passing over towards the palmar aspect of these lateral strands we reach the palmar surface of the palmar aponeurosis. The lateral borders of the anchors seem very impressive from this approach and they are in fact the lateral borders of the palmar aponeurosis. In the palmar dissection this border is found deeply placed in the ulnar niche of the preparation and this deep layer is covered by superficial layers of the palmar aponeurosis (Fig. 7.5).

Returning to our dissection we will again examine the skin anchor. In Figure 7.4 we have seen a continuation of this system passing away from the skin in a dorsal direction, represented by a flat band having a free proximal border and maintaining a somewhat sagittal position.

The ulnar flexor compartment wall can be looked upon as a septum derived from the palmar aponeurosis. The ulnar wall has a free

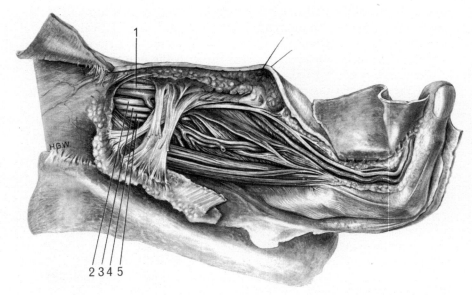

Fig. 7.6 (T. 1785; neg. 24792). Dissection
of the hypothenar area. The ulnar nerve
and vessels are partly hidden from view
by the palmaris brevis and by fibrous
anchors from the abductor fascia. 1. =
branch superficial to ulnar artery, partly
joining the branch to the fourth interspace
and partly anastomosing with the median
nerve; 2. = branch to the fourth interspace;
3. = branch to digit V; 4. = deep branch;
5. = hypothenar branch.

proximal border as pictured in Figure 7.5 and what also can be seen
in this drawing is that transverse layers of the palmar aponeurosis
contribute to the formation of this wall.

A few strands of the ulnar anchors, forming the most lateral border,
continue distally to participate in the formation of the 'languette' of
the little finger which ends just beyond the distal palmar crease.
Access to the subcutaneous area distal to the skin anchor is impaired
by fibrous strands running between the hypothenar compartment wall
and the skin. Nerve branches are seen, again seeking their way
towards the skin along the ulnar border of the aponeurosis.

We think it useful to pinpoint a few of the phenomena visible in
Figure 7.5. The exploration has been carried out considerably further
in 7.5 than in 7.4, particularly with regard to the flexor tendon
compartment wall. We wish especially to emphasize the existence of
the free distal border of the flexor retinaculum, which can be traced
as the proximal continuation of the inner border of the superficial
opponens itself; it is the innermost muscle in the drawing. We also
see the proximal free border of the ulnar compartment wall. Between
these two borders the flexor compartment lies open, which means
that we can explore the volar superficial arch of the hand and the
division of the superficial ulnar nerve and also the deep branch of the
volar arch. This artery runs on the peritendineal layer of the ulnar
bursa. This foramen can be located in the drawing by means of the
branches from the superficial volar arch.

Another point which deserves our attention relates to the ulnar
flexor tendon compartment wall just distal to the remarkable
bifurcated ligament where the transverse system of the palmar
aponeurosis contributes to this wall, while fibres from the wall are
seen to radiate towards the skin instead of continuing into this
transverse layer.

At their point of exit from the palmar aponeurosis compartment
the tendons are still enclosed in their peritendineal sleeve which can
be locally isolated from the compartment wall. More distally the
peritendineal wall becomes transformed into a strong fibrous tunnel

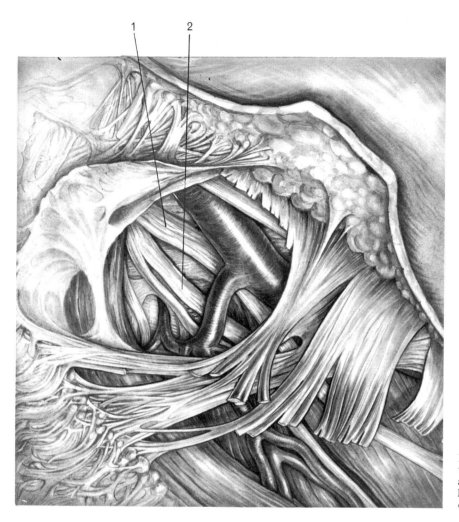

Fig. 7.7. (T. 1788; neg. 24795). Detail of the proximal hypothenar area. The oblique abductor fascia anchors are clearly visible here. 1.=branches to interspace IV and digit V; 2.=deep branch.

at metacarpophalangeal level. On the ulnar side this fibrous tunnel is firmly anchored to the ulnar sesamoid bone. Just beyond the tendon sheath in the drawing the common digital artery, the volar nerves and the lumbrical can all be seen.

3. The third dissection was carried out again on a left hand (Figs. 7.6, 7.7, 7.8 and 7.9).

This dissection extended into the hypothenar muscular area and included the topography of the ulnar nerve and artery. The main results will be given in the next section and here we will limit ourselves to a few observations on the fibrous arrangement of the region. As in previous dissections we see fibrous extensions from the abductor fascia, reinforced by palmaris brevis fibres, joining the palmar aponeurosis on its lateral border and passing to the skin (Figs. 7.6 and 7.7).

The midway skin anchor was also found in this preparation and could be identified as such because of its distinct continuation into the distal portion of the ulnar flexor tendon compartment wall. The proximal origin of this anchor could be traced in the extensions from

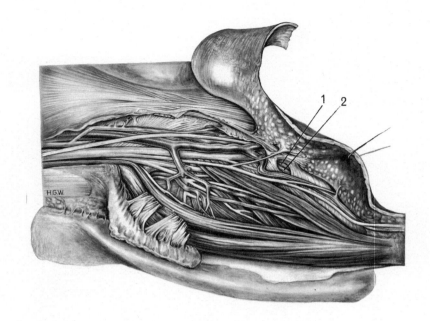

Fig. 7.8 (T. 1786; neg. 24793). The palmaris brevis has been divided so that the hypothenar muscular area can be thoroughly explored. This includes the ramifications of the ulnar nerve and artery. The most radial branch of the ulnar nerve passes over the ulnar artery. The ulnar skin anchorage of the palmar aponeurosis and the ulnar flexor compartment wall emanating from it are quite visible. Notice the abductor minimus bundle passing along the pisiform and also the bundles from the opponens layer that join the abductor. 1.=n.ulnaris; 2.=tendon V.

the abductor fascia which are reinforced by distally deviating fibres of the palmaris brevis. However, before dealing with this point in more detail, it is perhaps useful to record the exploration of the ulnar root of the palmar aponeurosis.

It is obvious that exploration of the ulnar nerve-vessel bundle leads to the ulnar root of the palmar aponeurosis, derived from the pisiform-hamulus column. We decided to expose the ulnar root more extensively than in previous preparations by dividing the palmaris brevis. We had also made an access to the palmar aponeurosis by removing the overlying skin in the palmar triangle. This made it possible to trace the proximal strand of the palmaris brevis in the niche between the palmar aponeurosis and the flexor retinaculum where it ultimately fuses with the retinaculum. We could establish now that the ulnar root (of considerable extent in this specimen) reinforces the palmar aponeurosis as a deep layer to it (Figs. 7.8 and 7.9). The dissection leads easily to the more distal part of the palmaris brevis and to extensions of the abductor fascia which join the tendinous layer of the brevis. Both structures blend medially and distally with the palmar aponeurosis, the latter already reinforced by the ulnar root.

It is obvious that a dense interweaving of tissues takes place between this transverse-longitudinal palmaris brevis tendon plate and the palmar aponeurosis. This blending of the two systems provides a lateral skin anchorage in the formation of which both palmar aponeurosis and the mediodistally running strands in the palmaris brevis plate participate. This skin anchor is located just distal to the flexor retinaculum. A remarkable feature seen in this preparation is that this skin anchor is used as the site of origin for opponens bundles. It can further be seen that a strand of fibres continues distally through this skin anchor to become inserted into the skin slightly distal to the midway skin anchor. The latter is recognized as such because the ulnar flexor compartment wall arises from this spot in a dorsal direction. The ulnar wall of the flexor

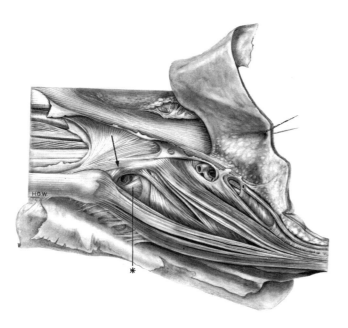

Fig. 7.9 (T. 1787; neg. 24794). The same area as in Fig. 7.8 after removal of the ulnar nerve and vessels. The dissection at this stage gives a clear picture of the hypothenar muscular area, of the flexor retinaculum and of the medial bundle of the pisometacarpal ligament, the latter passing in front of the hamulus (*). Notice the anchorage into the skin of the ulnar border of the palmar aponeurosis and the ulnar flexor compartment wall. Both the deep and superficial opponens layer are visible here. The arrow indicates the ulnar root of the palmar aponeurosis.

compartment can be identified in the drawings by means of its proximal free border.

The Hypothenar Muscular Compartment including the Ulnar Nerve and Artery

The topography of the ulnar nerve and artery can be read from the drawings of the specimen reported in dissection no. 3 of the first section of this paragraph.

Figure 7.6 represents the first stage of this dissection. The abductor has been drawn aside to give access to the inside of the hypothenar. The deep branch of the ulnar nerve can be traced between the two opponens layers, which assists the recognition of the hamulus ossis hamati in the drawing because the superficial opponens originates from the tip of this process. The nerves for the hypothenar muscles branch from the deep ulnar nerve (Fig. 7.7). This arrangement is better seen in the second stage of the dissection (Fig. 7.8) in which the palmaris brevis and the fibrous anchors from the abductor fascia have been removed.

The superficial ulnar nerve passes over the hamulus. Its branch to the ulnar side of the little finger remains external to the distal ulnar wall of the flexor compartment. A second branch of the ulnar nerve runs separately from the main bundle for the fourth interspace over the carpal area towards the midhand, which partly establishes an anastomosis with the median nerve, while the remainder joins the main superficial branch for the fourth interspace.

In the next stage of the dissection (Fig. 7.9) the nerves and vessels have been removed to enable us to see the ligament system as it radiates from the pisiform. It appears that the pisohamate ligament runs inwards from the pisiform as an extremely strong bundle and as this ligament has a considerable dorsopalmar extension it has a distinct distal aspect and a deep tunnel is formed with the innermost pisometacarpal bundle that leads along the root of the hamulus towards the triquetrum-hamatum joint.

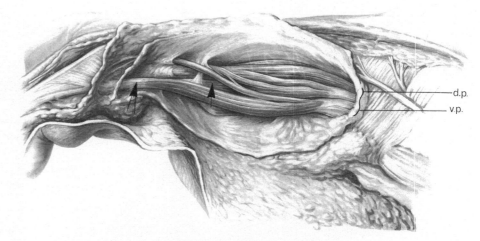

Fig. 7.10 (T. 1056; neg. 16313). Dissection of the hypothenar muscles. Below the wing tendon a bundle appears indicated in Fig. 7.5 by an arrow. d.p. = dorsal abductor portion; v.p. = volar abductor portion; arrow = the bundle to the base of the phalanx. The upper border of this bundle is a tiny bundle from the dorsal belly passing to the wing; double arrow = wing tendon.

The Hypothenar Muscular Area

The muscular compartment has been explored by blunt dissection in a number of specimens, two of which have been shown here (Figs. 7.4, 7.5, 7.10 and Figs. 7.6, 7.8, 7.9). As the situation in these two specimens is virtually the same we will restrict ourselves to a closer analysis in particular of only one of the preparations (Figs. 7.4, 7.5, 7.10). A major division in the hypothenar area is effected by the existence of a fairly strong intermuscular fascia lying between the opponens and the other hypothenar muscles (Fig. 7.5). However, not only does this fascia become quite thin distally but we see that a muscular portion of considerable size (Fig. 7.5; ○) leaves the bed of the opponens to join the abductor group as it passes to the phalanx. This muscle belly is reinforced by smaller bellies from the abductor division (Fig. 7.5; arrow) to form a common tendon that becomes inserted into the base of the phalanx, on its palmar aspect. For this reason and also because it originates from the hamulus this muscle could be called a flexor digiti minimi brevis. However, the palmar part of the abductor proper hardly differs in position from the flexor and therefore we wonder whether the distinction of a flexor proper is sensible. The abductor division will be explored further. Two bellies can be distinguished at the origin of the pisiform, a palmar and a dorsal; they have separate tendons of insertion. The existence of bridges between the two main bellies makes the situation somewhat complicated, but we believe that the following account covers the situation adequately.

In the origin of the abductor proper we have described two major divisions: (1) palmar and (2) dorsal (Fig. 7.10). The major part of the *palmar portion* (1) continues its way distally towards the ulnar wing of the extensor assembly of the fifth finger. A deeper greater part of this tendon detaches from it and is inserted into the phalangeal base while the smaller part only is found to pass into the wing. This

wing tendon is reinforced by a tiny bundle from the *dorsal portion* (2)
which can just be located in the drawing. The wing is reinforced
further by a tiny bundle from the main wing tendon that detaches
from the dorsal aspect of this muscle and is inserted into the dorsal
aspect of the wing. A number of insertions into the phalangeal base
can be seen (Fig. 7.10). By repeated delaminations of the transverse
lamina the tendons become incorporated into pericapsular layers and
become inserted into the phalangeal base. The insertions are found
along the lateral aspect of the phalangeal base as far as the palmar
ulnar tubercle. The major tendon inserting into the phalangeal base
is derived from the dorsal muscle portion and it is reinforced by a
twin bundle from the adjacent part of the volar portion of the muscle.

The other major insertion into the phalanx is derived from the
muscle bundle originating in the hamulus, with the superficial
opponens. This bundle is reinforced by a deep bundle from the palmar
portion of the abductor. These bundles are visible in Figure 7.5
(arrow), the latter bundle is just visible underneath the wing tendon
in Figure 7.10. A very strong tendon is formed which is inserted into
the ulnopalmar aspect of the phalanx proximal to the insertion of the
phalangeal tendon derived from the wing tendon.

A tiny, flat, deeply placed tendon arises from the dorsal abductor
portion, where it borders the opponens fascia. In Figure 7.10 the
small bundle is just visible at the upper border of the muscle. This
tendon disappears in pericapsular layers as it is covered by the main
dorsal phalangeal tendon. It extends towards the palmar side below
the tendons described. The phalangeal tendon derived from the wing
tendon has already been mentioned. A tendon emerges from a small
muscle bundle on the palmar aspect of the palmar abductor portion
which becomes part of capsular layers on the palmar side of the joint.

Figures 7.6, 7.8 and 7.9 show that the situation in the hypothenar
of the other specimen is closely similar to that found in the specimen
just described. In this specimen we have to observe that one abductor
bundle runs along the pisiform bone into the lower arm. The general
arrangement of the muscles in this specimen is given in the description
that follows and can be seen in the drawings.

Flexor bundles originate from the hamulus, with the superficial
opponens layer, and distally abductor bundles from the pisiform
merge with bundles originating from the hamulus (Fig. 7.9). The
division of the abductor proper into the two major portions occurs
again in this second preparation. The main palmar portion shifts
proximally along the pisiform into the lower arm. A conspicuous
phenomenon in this preparation concerns an additional origin of the
opponens from the midway skin anchorage.

Summary of the Ulnar Approach

An analysis of serial sections of the subcutaneous hypothenar area
has proved to be valuable for its micro-exploration. It seems advisable
to define some structural and spatial features peculiar to this area,
which are indispensable to a competent exploration. The features we
wish to list are (1) the pisiform skin anchor, (2) the ulnar root of the
palmar aponeurosis, including extensions from the abductor fascia
and (3) the skin anchorage on the inner side of the hypothenar space.
The ulnar nerve and vessels can be explored proximal to the

palmaris brevis. Passing below the pisiform skin anchor a spacious adipose body has to be removed. Then the flexor retinaculum and the ulnar root of the palmar aponeurosis (derived from the pisiform-hamulus column) can be traced distal to the pisiform. By gently displacing the abductor we can explore the deep fissure lateral to the hamulus, where special attention should be given to the deep branch of the ulnar nerve and the artery of the hypothenar muscles and the pisometacarpal ligament. It is obvious that this exploration enables the tip of the hamulus and the pisohamate bundle to be located with precision. The ulnar root of the palmar aponeurosis can be made more widely accessible by severing the pisiform skin anchorage. We could establish the extension of this ulnar root as the deep layer of the palmar aponeurosis. The skin anchorages are conspicuous along the inner border of the hypothenar both in cross-section and in dissection.

Palmaris brevis bundles which diverge distally have been seen to merge either with distally running fibrous strands originating from the abductor fascia and from the ulnar root of the palmar aponeurosis or with a distal extension of the carpal subcorial strata. It is these distally running strands that blend with the lateral border of the palmar aponeurosis (it may be as a deep layer) that account for the marked skin anchorages. Lateral extensions from the palmaris brevis plate to the skin do exist, as we have seen both on dissection and under the microscope.

A most conspicuous skin anchor is the so-called 'midway' anchor lying just distal to the palmaris brevis, from which site a strong lamina extends into the depth of the hand as the ulnar wall of the flexor compartment. This septum is firmly anchored to the volar crest of the fifth metacarpal bone. In this septum we have been able to trace longitudinal fibres derived from the palmar aponeurosis or its ulnar root.

The ulnar side of the carpal tunnel has a free distal border which represents the free distal border of the fibrous continuity of the hamulus. The ulnar artery will form the volar carpal arch at the distal border of the flexor retinaculum. It gives an ulnar branch which joins the most ulnar branch of the volar ulnar nerve and a deep arterial branch which passes round the ulnar bursa of the flexor tendon on its way to the deep palmar space. It is obvious that the deep nerve and the deep artery meet just at the distal border of the carpal canal, the nerve having passed between the two opponens layers and the artery having rounded the flexor tendons. The distal segment of the ulnar compartment wall extends from the 'midway' skin anchor and passes between palmar IV and the opponens layer to form an intramuscular septum, which is inserted later into the fifth metacarpal. In other words palmar IV, lying lateral to the ulnar wall of the carpal canal at proximal levels, becomes incorporated within the deep midpalmar area, as do the nerve and artery.

The hypothenar muscular area has been explored. The two layered opponens can be easily identified with the deep ulnar nerve passing in between. The flexor digiti minimi arises from the bed of the opponens, and is reinforced by bundles from the palmar abductor portion and is inserted into the base of the phalanx. The abductor can be divided into palmar and dorsal portions. The wing tendon arises from the more palmar portion, which also gives origin to a

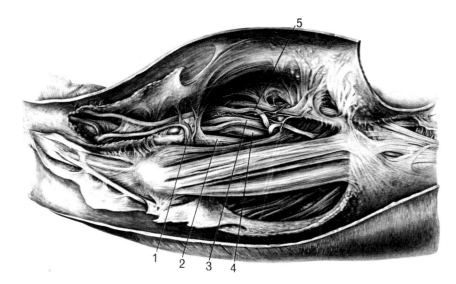

Fig. 7.11 (T. 1496; neg. 21706). Radial exploration. Muscles of the thenar eminence: the abductor, opponens and flexor. The motor branch of the median nerve. At the thenar base we see the palmaris longus which is partly anchored into the thenar base and partly passes the eminence to continue its way into the palmar aponeurosis. The access to the palmar surface of the palmar aponeurosis is shielded locally by extensions from the palmar aponeurosis into the thenar skin. The branch of the median nerve to the lateral side of the thumb and the twin branch of the same nerve to the adjacent sides of thumb and index are in the field of observation. 1.=radial artery for thumb; 2.=thumb flexor tendon; 3.=common digital nerve for first interspace; 4.= tendon for index with lumbrical I; 5.=radial digital nerve for thumb.

phalangeal tendon which becomes inserted into the ulnopalmar aspect of the phalanx just distal to the flexor brevis.

2. THE RADIAL APPROACH

This approach begins with an incision along the lateral side of thumb and thenar eminence (Fig. 7.11). Allowing for the fact that the palmar aponeurosis, with its various fascicles, is inserted into the the subcorial layers of the thenar, we decided to enter the hand by passing above and across the thenar musculature. It is obvious that this approach will lead straight into the flexor tendon compartment below the palmar aponeurosis. The dissection was carried out both superficially and deep to the flexor tendons. Ramifications of the median nerve and of the superficial carpal arch are found in the superficial space. The following structures are shown in the drawing made of this dissection (1) the recurrent branch of the median nerve for the thenar musculature, (2) the radial volar branch of the thumb and (3) the volar nerves for the adjacent sides of the thumb and the index finger originating from a common stem.

The artery for the radial side of the thumb can be followed proximally for a short distance only as it disappears in the depth of the preparation beneath the flexor pollicis longus. The radial volar artery of the index and the ulnar branch of the thumb arise from the superficial carpal arch in a common stem.

The flexor tendon of the thumb is in view and the first lumbrical muscle lying next to the flexor sheath as it leaves the index flexor profundus, can be brought into view. The skin anchorages of the palmar aponeurosis, seen in Figure 7.14, are viewed here from their inferior aspect and related to the proximal radial anchor. The palmaris longus tendon is exposed in the wrist area; it is anchored into the base of the thenar and extends into the palmar aponeurosis. The thenar musculature has been explored as far as possible. In the drawing are represented the abductor pollicis which is a well developed muscle in this specimen consisting of as many as three distinct bellies,

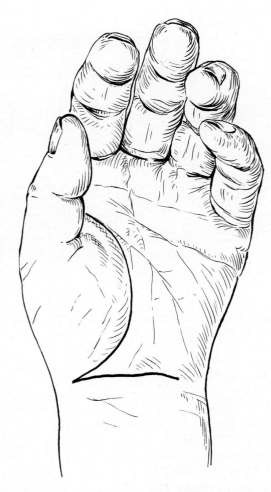

Fig. 7.12 (T. 1421; neg. 21142). This drawing shows the incisions which gave access to the palmar triangle and it may serve as a key to Figs. 7.13, 7.14 and 7.15.

the opponens pollicis and the superficial belly of the flexor pollicis brevis.

3. THE PALMAR APPROACH

The Palmar Triangle

In this section the results are presented of a dissection of the palmar aponeurosis and related structures and of an exploration of structures below this fibrous system, e.g. vessels and nerves, as far as they may be separated by blunt dissection and fibrous strands comprising this system. An incision has been made through the thenar crease and along the distal carpal crease to reflect a skin flap ulnarwards (Fig. 7.12). Progress is arrested naturally at the distal palmar crease by very strong skin anchorages which arise from the longitudinal strands of the palmar aponeurosis, so preventing the skin flap from being reflected further than shown in Figure 7.13. Inspection of the palmar aponeurosis had therefore to be carried out from different angles. In Figure 7.14 the palmar and radial aspects have been brought into view. The ulnar relations require a more radial angle of observation (Fig. 7.15).

We have dissected and reflected the skin of the thenar eminence

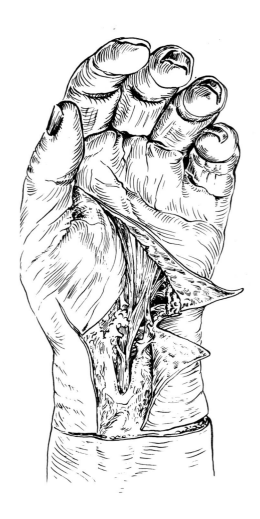

Fig. 7.13 (T. 1276; neg. 19075). The skin has been dissected from the palmar triangle. An additional area at the wrist has been included in the dissection.

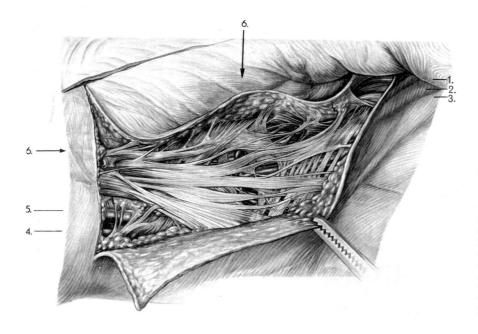

Fig. 7.14 (T. 1447; neg. 21200). Palmar dissection. View towards the radial side. Insertion of deep palmar aponeurosis layers and of more superficial layers into the thenar skin. Notice the convergence of bundles forming the radial flexor compartment wall. At the level of the arrow on the right side: the interdigital space II–III. 1.=artery (for the radial side of the index); 2.=lumbrical (for the radial side of the index); 3.=nerve (for the radial side of the index); 4.=superficial branch n.ulnaris without branch for ulnar aspect of digit V; 5.=a.ulnaris; 6.=the branch of the volar superficial arch for the radial side of the index and for the ulnar side of the thumb. Below it we see the tendon of the index and the nerves of the first interspace.

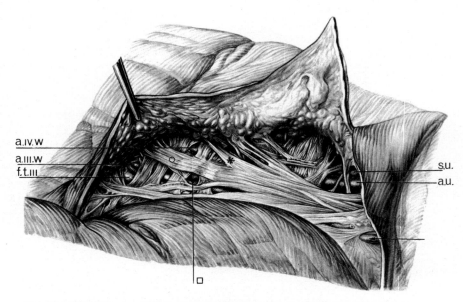

Fig. 7.15 (T. 1490; neg. 21701). Palmar dissection after incision along the thenar eminence and a transverse incision over the wrist. Deep view into the ulnar niche of the dissection field. The languettes to the ring finger (○) and to the little finger are visible (*). Note the proximal roots of the palmar aponeurosis septa, the ulnar skin anchorages and the palmaris brevis. s.u. = superficial branch of the ulnar nerve; a.u. = ulnar artery; a.IV.W = common digital artery of fourth webspace; f.t.III = flexor tendon of third finger; a.III.W = common digital artery of third webspace; □ = proximal border of septum; arrow = volar branch of radial artery; r.r.p. = ramus radiopalmaris.

(Fig. 7.14) for the short distance that the anchorage of palmar aponeurosis strands into the thenar skin would allow. The major portion of the superficially visible palmar aponeurosis is a continuation of the palmaris longus tendon and an ulnar strand of the aponeurosis takes its origin from subcorial layers in the carpal region. Part of the palmaris longus tendon is inserted into the base of the fibrofascial wall of the thenar compartment.

Starting at a proximal carpal base we will examine the extensions of the palmar aponeurosis and the various other structures which will be met with. Apart from the thenar anchorage of the palmaris longus described above, there are some strands, limited in size and strength, which are inserted proximally into the thenar skin. A much stronger strand of fibres inserted into the thenar skin about halfway along the thenar crease is derived from a deeper layer of the palmar aponeurosis. This system is composed of obliquely running fibres which can be traced both into the flexor retinaculum and as far as their insertions into the thenar skin, receiving local reinforcing strands derived from the palmaris longus. From this oblique fibre system more longitudinally running fibres merge distally with longitudinal palmar aponeurosis strands. These markedly strong fascicles are seen to be inserted into the thenar skin, while the most distal extension of the system can be seen to form the radial wall of the flexor compartment. This distal part of the radial system is again reinforced by transverse fibres from the transverse layer of the palmar aponeurosis. The radial wall of the flexor compartment has the index lumbrical and the volar digital nerve and artery running along it externally. This radial compartment wall has more fibrous contributions that have been explored and reproduced in this drawing. We can distinguish two more strands, each arising from the thenar skin. One of these is a long fibre system that can be explored by passing at the radial side of the longitudinal strand just mentioned. Then we find fibres that can be followed proximally as far as the insertion of the oblique layer into the thenar skin where they are inserted; it is a very strong system passing distally below the palmar aponeurosis fascicle and merging with it into the radial compartment wall. The other strand, so actually the third one, is shorter. This one is a flat band originating from within the thenar skin area close to the point of insertion of the longitudinal strand at the bend of the thenar crease. This is also a remarkably strong band. Fibrous extensions arising from the thenar skin and passing along the outer side of the lumbrical, the nerve and artery are also present, but they could not be shown in this drawing. The radial anchorages of the palmar fibrous system have now been fully described.

There is only a tiny longitudinal strand from the palmar aponeurosis that continues its way in a distal direction, running in the axis of the index finger. A fairly broad band represents the fascicle for the middle finger and fascicles or languettes of the fourth and fifth fingers.

By carefully separating the longitudinal fibres from each other we see a conspicuous phenomenon. The fibres of a deeper layer run obliquely in an ulnodistal direction and seem to belong to the same layer as the radial oblique system. It should not be interpreted that the one necessarily arises from the other, since our observations support the assumption that this deep layer arises from the flexor retinaculum below the radial oblique layer and closely adherent to it and that it almost exclusively reinforces the languettes of the fourth and fifth fingers.

We were able to explore various nerves and branches of the volar arterial arch when passing between various fascicles of the palmar aponeurosis and related structures. Another exploration (Fig. 7.5) showed that the ulnar nerve and vessels are directly accessible from the subcutaneous space proximal to the palmaris brevis. Here we have exposed the superficial branches of both the nerve and artery and we followed their branches between the fascicles of the palmar aponeurosis.

We have explored the artery and nerves for both the space between the index and middle fingers and between the middle and fourth fingers. It is also possible to trace and isolate the radial digital nerve for the index between the radial skin anchors, although it could not be shown in this drawing. The nerve has been shown in this drawing at the base of the index just volar to the lumbrical. Proximally this nerve can be followed to a stem in common with the ulnar digital nerve of the thumb. This common digital nerve is detached proximally from the median complex. The radial volar artery of the index can be followed in the same space from where it originates from the volar arch.

A final point for consideration concerns the formation of partitions derived from the palmar aponeurosis, which are obviously extremely difficult to visualize because they penetrate into the depth of the preparation. We have checked the ulnar partition of the index tendon, the radial and the ulnar walls of the middle finger tendon and the radial and ulnar walls of the ring finger tendon.

The formations are quite typical. They start with proximally concave, sickle-like, free borders and longitudinal fibres of the palmar aponeurosis are seen to enter these structures. The sickle of the ulnar wall of the index tendon is shown in this drawing. The ulnar partition of the index tendon is composed of fibres which pass deep to the most proximal transverse fibres and are in relation to the index tendon. Another deep bundle aids in the formation of a partition wall on the ulnar side of the middle finger.

The ulnar view of this palmar exploration (Fig. 7.15) requires only a short description. In this drawing it is obvious that both dissection and drawing were made before the additional wrist area was prepared. The important points concern structures which were present in the exploration of the subcutaneous hypothenar area.

As found in the 'ulnar approach' of this preparation, the main contribution from the pisiform area to the palmar aponeurosis passes superficial to the ulnar nerve-vessel bundle; as in the transverse series such radiations originate from the abductor minimus fascia.

It seems appropriate now to report further on the palmar exploration. First let us be sure that the ulnar border of the palmaris longus does not continue as the ulnar border of the palmar aponeurosis. We have seen contributions from a subcorial layer close to the palmaris longus tendon and fibres originating from a deeper position spiralling round the lateral border to form a new lateral border for the palmar aponeurosis.

It is evident that this approach will bring the palmaris brevis into view. The tendinous sheet of this structure passes below the palmar aponeurosis, but not without dense interweaving with the deeper layers of this aponeurosis. We also see that the palmaris brevis layer is occupied by somewhat irregularly placed fibrofascial strands which originate either deep to the palmar aponeurosis or from subcorial strata in the region of the pisiform skin anchor. Other fibrous strands (palmaris brevis-like) are seen to emerge from below the palmar aponeurosis and instead of joining the palmaris brevis layer proper they are inserted directly into the skin, somewhere along the inner border of the hypothenar eminence.

The so-called 'midway' skin anchor of the hypothenar area can be brought into view in this palmar approach by penetrating deeply into the ulnar niche of the field of preparation. It is obvious that both the proximal and the distal continuities of this anchor can be explored better by the ulnar approach. On the other hand, it is possible to see here other continuities into the ulnar wall of the flexor compartment. We can establish that the two strands of the palmar aponeurosis shown in Figure 7.15 are for the fourth and fifth fingers. A small arterial branch skirts the ulnar side of the fascicle for the fifth finger.

On the ulnar side of this arterial branch is a strand of fibres seen in the drawing to be inserted into the skin; this same strand contributes to the ulnar flexor compartment wall and so joins the fibres which arise from the skin anchor; this is shown in Figures 7.3 and 7.5 and can be seen here just proximal to the bundle mentioned above. The palmaris brevis is found here again proximal to this anchor. Longitudinal fibres from the palmaris brevis join this skin anchor and there are also palmaris brevis fibres which are inserted into the skin in an ulnar direction.

same angles in the middle and third phalanges yields a measure of the longitudinal deviation. Holcomb *et al.* made an analysis of the phenomenon during flexion and extension in the proximal interphalangeal joint. They made it clear that the cause of deviation might be found either in tilt or in coronal deviation of the phalangeal trochlea. Tilt is a rotation of the axis of the trochlea in a plane perpendicular to the shaft; coronal deviation is a deviation of the mechanical axis of the joint from the mediolateral anatomical axis occurring in the coronal plane. Holcomb *et al.* were able to demonstrate a significant radial deviation in the fifth finger during flexion of the proximal interphalangeal joint. The geometrical analysis made it probable that this deviation was due mainly to coronal deviation, a conclusion that in its turn is strongly supported by Shiino's measurements of the first phalanx of the fifth finger, the mean value of the angle between shaft and trochlea being $\bar{x} = 95 \cdot 16$; s.d. $2 \cdot 16$, the angle being measured on the radial side.

The tendency to ulnar divergence in the proximal interphalangeal joint of the index (in particular the right index) tallies with the measurements of Shiino in his 30 individuals who found the angle between shaft and trochlea to be $\bar{x} = 87 \cdot 63$; s.d. $2 \cdot 74$. However small this divergence in these two respective joints may be, it should be realized that in both the index and the minimus this divergence fits an efficient way of gripping. As for the other fingers, Shiino's data regarding deviations in the extended position of medius and ring finger and those of Holcomb on divergence in flexion, suggest that these fingers on the average do not show marked deviations.

Interossei, Thenar and Hypothenar

Interossei, lumbricals, thenar and hypothenar muscles together constitute the intrinsic musculature of the hand.

Interossei

We presented a thorough analysis of the structure of interossei in Chapter 3. Salsbury (1937) made important observations on interosseal anatomy, based on dissections, the main results of which we were able to confirm (Landsmeer, 1955). Salsbury's findings touched mainly upon whether or not phalangeal and/or wing tendons occur in various interossei. Serial analyses, as presented for dorsal IV, III and II (Landsmeer, 1965, 1966), showed both the inner structure of the muscles and their relations, particularly in the metacarpophalangeal areas. The individual specificity of the interossei does not prevent the distinction between dorsal and volar interossei from remaining perfectly valid. Differences presented within each group are quite understandable on the basis of a common structural and spatial denominator.

We wish to add here a few remarks regarding the close connection between the arrangement in the metacarpophalangeal region and the structure of the interossei. The transverse laminae play a key-role in guiding the interossei tendons, either into the extensor assembly or to the phalangeal tubercles. Formation of multiple tendons in interossei is a common feature and it may be accompanied by the formation of an intramuscular septum. A marked form of an intramuscular septum is regularly found in dorsal II and in dorsal IV and it effects the division of these muscles into phalangeal and wing portions. Distally such a septum merges into the transverse lamina. We should also mention both the anchorage of interossei to the transverse intermetacarpal ligament and the merging of phalangeal tendons with the outer anchors of the volar plate. The concept of the transverse laminae guiding the respective interossei tendons to their sites of insertion was duly considered by Lewis (1965), in a study of the evolution of the interossei muscles of the primate hand.

Thenar and Hypothenar (*general remarks*)

It can be seen in the cross-sections that the formation of a carpal tunnel, which accommodates the digital flexors, creates space for the origin of the marginal intrinsics; while the hamulus, the bony stronghold of the carpal tunnel, is of equal importance as the site of origin of intrinsic muscles. In this connection it might be useful to recall what has been said about the different relations of the carpal eminences to the carpal tunnel. The hamulus is virtually a bony wall of the carpal tunnel, the radial wall being entirely fibrous and attached secondarily, by what we have termed the radial root of the flexor retinaculum, to the scaphoid and trapezium. This situation tallies well with embryological observations made by Čihák (1972), who found that in early stages the flexor retinaculum is anchored to the hamulus, while radially it *ends freely* in the mesenchyme. In view of the considerable ulnar extension of both opponens and flexor pollicis brevis into the flexor retinaculum, it is clear that the hamulus also provides a stronghold for the origin of the thenar muscles.

Thenar

After these preliminary remarks we may now briefly review the position of the various muscles of the two eminences, the thenar and hypothenar. The precarious path of thenar terminology has been traced back by Day and Napier (1961) in a very careful manner. Moreover, they dissected the thenar musculature in a great number of hands and invariably found a definite connective tissue plane between the oblique head of the adductor and the deep head of the flexor pollicis brevis, which made it possible to distinguish this deep part of the muscle in those cases (9 out of 65) where this deep head, either partly or in its entirety, joined the adductor to insert into the ulnar sesamoid. In the majority of their material (53 out of 65 cases) the deep head joined the superficial one to insert into the radial sesamoid. In 3 out of 65 cases the deep head was absent.

On viewing the insertion of the adductor and the flexor brevis a conspicuous difference can be noticed in that a large part of the adductor tendon passes dorsal to the ulnar sesamoid and towards the base of the phalanx, while in the flexor brevis the radial sesamoid absorbs practically all its fibres. It is perhaps useful to mention that the radial artery and the deep ulnar nerve do not use the same opening in the adductor, while distal to the passage of the artery over the second metacarpal, another small bundle of the adductor takes origin. The opponens pollicis becomes gradually replaced by the superficial head of the flexor brevis, the latter originating from the flexor retinaculum by two discrete heads on either side of the opponens.

The abductor pollicis need hardly be commented upon, except perhaps to establish that only a small portion of its fibres continues into the wing of the assembly.

Hypothenar

In the hypothenar area the abductor holds a prominent place owing to its conspicuous internal arrangement. This muscle, originating from the pisiform and from the adjacent reinforced fascial layers, extends in front of the pisiform and the pisometacarpal ligaments, the latter converging towards the base of the fifth and fourth metacarpals. It is a muscle of conspicuous structural refinement as can be seen in cross-sections and in microdissection. The opponens is a two-layered muscle arising from the hamulus. The superficial layer may give rise to a muscular bundle which extends to the phalangeal base, which is occasionally an individual muscle inserted via the volar plate into the phalangeal base, but more usually is entirely incorporated into the tendon system of the abductor. In the latter case the denomination of flexor brevis digiti V relates only to its origin from the hamulus and as identification in comparative anatomy. The course of the deep branch of the ulnar nerve, passing between the two opponens layers, has been meticulously described by Anderson (1894), the position of the ulnar nerve being a most important landmark in comparative anatomy.

2. THE PALMAR ANCHORING SYSTEM

Both Thomine (1965) and Stack (1973) made use of the serial sections of the Leiden collection; the former author investigated the digital fascia, the latter studied the palmar fascia, in particular its relations in the metacarpophalangeal region and its continuities in the finger.

A strict systemic description of the palmar aponeurosis seems to be basically incompatible with the nature of this structure and any schematic simplification of it should be referred to the integral system of the palmar aponeurosis, including its fascial continuities and its environmental relationships.

The explicit statement of Ferrarini (1936) on the independence of the palmar aponeurosis from both the thenar and hypothenar fasciae, which we basically confirm, is certainly not weakened by the presence of adhesions of palmaris longus fascicles to the thenar fascia and by adhesion of the hypothenar fascia either to the ulnar wall of the flexor compartment or to the fibrous anchors which are occasionally seen to originate from the abductor fascia and to merge into the palmar aponeurosis. The triangular extension of the tendon of the palmaris longus is heavily reinforced by fibres from the flexor retinaculum.

Deep intercrossing oblique fibres, previously observed by Legueu and Juvara (1892), represent the roots of the palmar aponeurosis in the flexor retinaculum. They have received too little attention so far, as has the so-called 'ulnar root' of the palmar aponeurosis, derived from the flexor carpi ulnaris-pisiform-hamate column. The fibres of this root could be traced into the lateral border of the palmar aponeurosis and into its deeper layers and thus may contribute to the oblique fibres. The radial and ulnar attachments of the palmar aponeurosis, also somewhat neglected in the literature, were thoroughly investigated in this study. The former, deep radiodistally directed fibres and superficial longitudinal fibres, provide anchorages for the thenar skin; from the thenar skin along the thenar crease fibrous radiations are found passing into the radial wall of the flexor compartment around and close to the flexor tendons of the index. A strong anchorage is found halfway along the hypothenar eminence in which the ulnar root of the aponeurosis plays an important part. From this site of anchorage fibres radiate to form the ulnar wall of the flexor compartment. The anchorage of the ulnar wall of the flexor tendon compartment to the skin and the attachment of the hypothenar fascia to this compartment wall, leads to the formation of what we have termed the 'carrefour hypothénarien'.

Evidence gathered from cross-sections and from dissections seems to warrant the conclusion that both the deep longitudinal fibres and the transverse system share in the formation of the compartments of the palmar aponeurosis, as is the case with both the radial and the ulnar wall of the flexor compartment. The languettes insert into the skin just beyond the distal palmar crease. The continuity between the palmar aponeurosis and the tendon sheath, which Maslieurat-Lagémard (1839) and Ferrarini (1936) alleged to exist, has always been a controversial point. Continuities between these structures do occur, but this does not prevent the two structures from being basically different. In common with Stack (1973) we wish to stress the fact that the tendon sheath and the synovial membrane are intimately attached to each other, with no areolar space intervening, which is in contrast to the situation between the compartment wall and synovial membrane. Horizontal and sagittal sections provide unequivocal evidence on this point.

The continuity of the palmar aponeurosis beyond the distal palmar crease remains difficult to assess. It seems beyond dispute that the palmar aponeurosis extends as a thin fascial layer over the metacarpophalangeal segment of the tendon sheath and also that strands of a more fibrous nature are included in these hoods, seeking their way via the lumbrical niches into the transverse intermetacarpal ligament and volar plates. At the exit of the palmar aponeurosis compartments, which is about the level of the distal palmar crease, the hoods are attached to the skin by means of fibres which can sometimes be traced as far as the transverse intermetacarpal ligament. Near the distal border of this ligament those fibres are often seen as perforating fibres, which means that they can be traced through this ligament into interossei tendons or derivatives thereof. The fibres also may find their way running free from the fascial hoods. The fascial covering of the sheath is quite thin in the webspace area.

Ferrarini (1936) emphasized that the natatorial ligament and the palmar aponeurosis are basically autonomous structures, a view which we are inclined to support. Junctions between the skin and deeper structures again occur at the level of the natatorial ligament, *in casu* the phalangeal base and this webspace region is relatively devoid of fibrous texture. Both tendon sheath and digital nerve and artery are accessible by simply removing fatty tissue and eventually the thin fascial covering of the sheath. Quite an important feature of this area is the transition of the metacarpophalangeal segment of the tendon sheath into the segment pertaining to phalanx I.

Fetal sections show the continuity of the metacarpophalangeal segment into a fascial layer, a continuity which includes the external anchor of the volar plate and as a result of which the tendon sheath segment of phalanx I is surrounded by a fascial hood holding the wing of the extensor assembly bilaterally. At the natatorial level this hood becomes considerably thickened; it attaches again to the phalangeal base and, with a layer derived from the natatorial ligament, it forms a duplicature for the digital nerve and artery. Distally this hood then loses its relation with the wing of the assembly and radiates in the lateral line of the finger, dorsal to the nerve and artery.

Horizontal and sagittal sections were unique in showing fibrous extensions passing into the digital band from the metacarpophalangeal area. Fibres from the transverse intermetacarpal ligament passing in front of the lumbrical proved to fit structurally into the distal fascial extension of the metacarpophalangeal segment of the sheath, including the volar plate and its distal outer anchor.

The palmar aponeurosis actually radiates into the same layer from which distal radiations are present. We should be reticent in accepting that direct fibrous continuities pass from the palmar aponeurosis into the finger. Apart from the most proximal origin of the digital band just described, the area between the distal palmar crease and the natatorial ligament is structured in such a way that full mobility of the joints is ensured. In the natatorial area the commissures between the fingers are again reinforced by fibrous systems. Thomine (1965) and Stack (1973) both paid considerable attention to this fibrous system.

In our point of view it is important to be fully cognisant with the transitions taking place within the tendon sheath which bear on the fascial constitution of the region.

A most illuminating and beautifully illustrated paper has been published recently by Bojsen *et al.* (1974). The authors describe the septa of the palmar aponeurosis in much detail, their relation to the flexor tendon sheaths, their deep anchorages and their proximal extensions. On the ulnar sides of the index and middle fingers the septa extend farthest in a proximal direction, without dividing the deep central compartment in two separate spaces.

3. THE FREE FINGER

The discussion leads easily onwards to the free fingers where considerable attention was paid to structural continuities, as in the metacarpophalangeal region. It could be shown that strong skin anchoring fibres emerge from the joints and that these anchoring systems are specifically arranged in each of the two joints. This specificity is not surprising in view of the marked differences in these respective joint regions. The extensor assembly is differently arranged in the respective finger joints and it is obvious that this bears directly on the interrelationship of the joints with their surroundings.

It may be helpful first to comment on the tendon sheath of the free finger. We should recall that the tendon sheath at phalanx I level is surrounded by the fascial hood derived from the sheath at metacarpophalangeal level. The fibrous spur of the natatorial system extends into the fingers as a fascial layer and so these two fascial layers form a nerve-vessel sheath, easily recognized in the first segment, the two layers fusing anterior to the sheath. We have mentioned that the so-called digital band is situated in this fascia, where it fuses dorsally with the nerve and artery.

Phalanx I segment of the sheath has a free distal border within the first interphalangeal segment, the latter merging as a thin fascial layer with the thick phalanx I segment. The first interphalangeal segment of the tendon sheath is characterized by the cruciform and annular ligaments. Proximally the cruciate ligaments are inserted into the shaft of the phalanx; distal to their crossing they blend with the volar plate of the joint, as does the annular ligament. Distally the sheath merges with the sheath segment of phalanx II, the latter presenting its proximal free border within the hood of the former. Differences between the two interphalangeal joints become manifest in the skin anchoring system, in the proximal attachment of the volar plates and in the proximal relations of the sheath segment related to the joint in question. The distal interphalangeal segment of the sheath passes proximally into the sheath segment of phalanx II and so does the volar plate of the distal interphalangeal joint. In contrast to this pattern, the sheath at the proximal interphalangeal level and the volar plate both show proximal anchorages into phalanx I. Both sagittal and horizontal series showed that the cruciate ligaments and the so-called 'proximal reins' of the volar plate are anchored into phalanx I, separately from the free distal border of the sheath segment of that phalanx. It seemed to us that the attachment of the flexor sublimis into the second phalanx absorbed the proximal roots (or anchors) of the volar plate which can be seen in the proximal interphalangeal joint.

Kuczynsky (1968) made mention of 'lower' fibres belonging to the lateral capsule of the proximal interphalangeal joint and pictured them with fibres of the cruciate part of the flexor sheath. He proved the importance of these fibres in preventing hyperextension of the proximal interphalangeal joint. In addition, we found proximal roots of the volar plate which are inserted into the proximal phalanx on the inner side of the sheath of phalanx I.

With regard to the skin anchoring system, it is obvious that what has been described by Cleland (1878) as the 'cutaneous ligaments' is a complex system derived partially from the joint ligaments and partially from the sheath and digital fascia. The joint derived systems have been thoroughly discussed. It is obvious that in the joint regions digital fasciae and tendon sheaths are fusing; the fascial extensions from the joint area are quite conspicuous. It is also important to pay due attention to the retroarticular vascular beds present in both interphalangeal joints and to their accessibility from the nerve-vessel bundle. The respective hila have been located precisely in relation to the sheath segments and in relation to the proximal extensions of the respective volar plates.

Lastly in cross-sections, the nail-bearing system of the terminal phalanx presents itself clearly. The vault of the nail is supported bilaterally by the fibrous strands running between the base of the third phalanx and its tuberosity. This arrangement places the third phalanx in a state of quasi-suspension, a state which may be of particular importance for the function of the subcutaneous pads of the distal segment.

The extensor assembly has been subjected to frequent and thorough structural and functional analysis so we may refrain for a while from discussing it again in detail. Moreover, the drawings give adequate evidence of the properties of this structure, as do the transverse sections, particularly those related to proximal interphalangeal levels.

4. SPACES IN THE HAND

It is obvious that the term 'space' cannot be applied unequivocally, and that its significance has to be evident from the context.

The Subcutaneous Hypothenar Space

We paid considerable attention to the subcutaneous hypothenar area because we became increasingly convinced that it has a significant position in the spatial arrangement of the human hand. In particular, the absence of a similar space in the thenar area led us to suppose that the relative positions of thumb and little finger have a bearing on the differences in development of these respective areas. In any examination of the subcutaneous hypothenar area the studies of both Kirk (1924) and Frohse (1906) should be mentioned. The first author discusses the subcutaneous volar pads in general and, while specifying the difference between the subcutaneous thenar and hypothenar areas, observes that the latter is larger and of greater thickness than the former. This author also stresses the importance of the palmaris brevis in maintaining the position of this space during the grasping action of the hand, so preventing it from being splayed round the ulnar margin.

Spaces in the Palm of the Hand

As a result of the formation of septa from the palmar aponeurosis the palm is conspicuously divided into compartments. At proximal levels of the midhand we tend to distinguish a single midpalmar space, which divides distalwards into seven compartments, or canals, alternately for the digital tendons and for the lumbricals and digital vessels. The septum on the ulnar side of the medius tendons is rather strongly developed and it extends for quite a distance in a proximal direction so that the midpalmar space becomes divided proximally into two parts. Towards the carpus an arterial pedicle approaches the flexor peritendineum from the deep carpal arch.

We believe that it goes too far to say there are as many potential spaces as there are muscular compartments. It might, however, be useful to distinguish the space of the adductor pollicis muscle as a gliding area below the midpalmar space: its extension being naturally that of the muscle itself.

Grodinsky and Holyoke (1941) locate palmar aponeurosis extensions in a superficial layer of the metacarpophalangeal tendon sheath, while we located them primarily as local reinforcements of the fascial hood around this sheath.

As for the synovial spaces it should be noticed that Kanavel (1925) described the synovial spaces around the superficial flexor tendons in the carpus, albeit that some of his figures are somewhat too simplified.

Spaces at the Dorsal Side of the Hand

In the dorsal aspect of the hand the situation is characterized by gliding fascial layers. In a previous paper (Landsmeer, 1955) the dorsal fasciae have been subjected to closer analysis and De Leeuw (1962), in his study of the dorsal carpal area, focused his attention particularly on the relations of the tendon sheath of the extensor carpi ulnaris. We gave due consideration to this point in our analysis of this area. In the forearm a gliding space exists between the subcutaneous fascia and the antebrachial fascia. The latter becomes reinforced in the carpus to provide the extensor retinaculum, which is in fact a too generalized term for the system of loops and rings of the extensor tendons. This layer runs freely over the sheath of the extensor carpi ulnaris. Distal to the carpal area this fascial layer becomes thinner and halfway along the metacarpus it fuses with the subcutaneous fascia, thus obliterating the dorsal gliding space. A new gliding space develops distal to the carpus between the intertendinous fascia and the distal extension of the extensor retinaculum, which may be designated the supratendineal fascia. On the dorsal side of the fingers the situation is virtually the same. Here too, the gliding space is located immediately above the extensor assembly. Between the fingers, the interdigital spur derived from the natatorial ligament merges into the subcutaneous layer, and vessels from the intermetacarpal spaces enter the subcutaneous layer here. Fascial attachments exist between the transverse laminae and the subcutaneous layer, with the result that the intermetacarpal spaces are sealed off distally. Over the metacarpus the supratendineal space closes towards the tendons of the fifth finger and radial to the tendons of the index finger. It is apparent that we adopted Anson's (1963) terminology for the layers and gliding spaces on the dorsal side of the hand. Kanavel (1925), Anson and Ashley (1940) and Grodinsky and Holyoke (1941) studied the spaces in the hand in general.

5. NERVES AND VESSELS

Nerves and vessels were not studied by us in a systemic way and we therefore have to refer to other sources.

Nerves of the Hand

Both regarding delicate descriptions of the nerves involved in innervation of the hand in its widest sense and continuous reference to the related literature, Hovelacque's (1927) monumental *Anatomie des nerfs craniens et rachidiens et du système grand sympathique* is unsurpassed. The cutaneous innervation on the palmar side is fairly constant, the musculo-cutaneous nerve and the palmar branch of the median nerve are involved in supplying the base of the thenar and a limited area of the palm respectively. The median nerve gives rise to seven of the volar digital nerves (collatéraux des doigts), the ulnar nerve to the remaining three and they all continue as far as the pulp of the third phalanx. The dorsal branches of the volar nerves play a conspicuous role in the innervation of the dorsal aspect of the fingers.

Dorsal branches are given off regularly from the digital branches of the median nerve, except those for the thumb. They arise proximally at the webspace and pass along the first phalanx, one then passes along the second phalanx and finally one branch goes through a passage covered by a ligament along the third phalanx. These latter branches reach the bed of the nail and it is important that these dorsal branches also occur in the thumb, explicitly described and illustrated by Brooks (1888): 'In three cases I traced particularly strong branches under the thumb nail, and found them ramifying in the bed of the nail. . . . The twigs from the median passed in these cases under cover of a ligamentous band, and wound round the ungual phalanx, keeping close to the bone, to reach the dorsal surface' (p. 467 l.c.).

The volar nerve on the ulnar side of the fifth finger never extends into the dorsal area, except for branches in the terminal pulp for the nailbed, the existence of which have not explicitly been denied. Dorsal extension of the radial nerve of the fifth finger rarely occurs, but it has been observed, and in our own material it can be seen in Figure 7.34.

The ulnar branch for the annularis regularly sends branches to the dorsal side. Where those dorsal branches from the volar sources occur, anastomosis with the dorsal nerves will possibly occur, which makes it feasible that, in spite of volar contribution, fibres of dorsal source may reach the nail (Hédon, 1889).

Although the volar pattern of distribution is fairly constant, anastomoses between ulnar and median nerves and the formation of elliptical loops, even into a plexiform arrangement, have been seen between the main branches and between branches of the nerve trees (Hartmann, 1887; Von Gehwolf, 1921). Moreover, the latter author clearly depicted the dorsal branches as springing from the main branch in the webspace, a feature sometimes neglected in later texts.

Distribution of the dorsal nerves has been described by Brooks (1888) in a finely illustrated paper and by Zander (1890). It proves that extension of the radial area at the expense of the ulnar field occurs far more frequently than the reverse. Apart from a shift of a borderline to the ulnar side the two areas may show considerable overlap, with or without anastomoses. With regard to the extension of dorsal branches over the fingers Brooks summarizes as follows: 'In five of the ten cases, the dorsal branches of the ulnar nerve were traced to the nail of the little finger, and, from the size of the nerves, they probably extended equally far in the other five cases also. In the thumb, as is well known, the branches of the radial regularly extend as far as the nail. In the index and ring fingers, I found that the dorsal nerves usually reached the second interphalangeal joint. In the middle finger the dorsal nerves generally extend only as far as the first interphalangeal articulation;' (p. 466 l.c.).

As for the pattern of nerve-endings in the skin, the reader is referred to a paper of Miller *et al.* (1958).

Another point of great interest relates to the anastomosis of the deep branch of the ulnar nerve with the median nerve, because this immediately affects the innervation of the thenar eminence. The course of the deep branch of the ulnar nerve between the two layers of the opponens has been reported in a paper by Anderson (1894) who provides a very appropriate drawing. This particular anastomosis was described by Riche (1897), and by Cannieu (1897) and ever since it has been known as the Cannieu–Riche anastomosis. Recently

Harness and Sekeles (1971) coined the term 'thenar ansa' for this anastomosis, which they found in 27 of 35 dissected hands. When we look at the innervation of the thenar eminence some difficulties arise with respect to the designation of the thenar musculature, a matter which was duly considered by Day and Napier (1961).

Brooks (1886) reports that innervation of the whole flexor brevis by the ulnar nerve was observed by him in 5 out of 30 cases. In the great majority the flexor brevis is innervated by both the median and ulnar nerves, but as Brooks did not distinguish the superficial and deep head of the flexor brevis pollicis, as had been advocated by Cruveilhier (1843), we cannot learn from his paper how median and ulnar nerves share their respective portions.

Day and Napier (1961) investigated the nerve supply in 40 specimens and their figures are quite suggestive that, while variation of the nerve supply is common, there is a tendency for the superficial head to be supplied by the median nerve (24 out of 30) and for the deep head to be supplied by the ulnar nerve (21 out of 24). It should be observed that in a minority of cases the ulnar extends its area as far as the superficial head, that the median nerve does so with respect to the deep head, in both cases either with exclusion of the other nerve or with its participation.

Electromyographic studies by Forrest (1967) and by Harness *et al.* (1974) showed a double innervation for the flexor pollicis brevis in about 75 per cent and for the opponens in 77 per cent of cases.

For an extensive bibliography concerning normal and anomalous innervation we refer to Mannerfelt (1964, 1966). Concerning the innervation of joints and of tendinous structures we refer to the older literature of Stopford (1921) and for more recent work to the important studies of Stilwell (1957) and Gray and Gardner (1965). Muscle spindles have been studied by Smith and Marcarian (1966) in interossei, and by Rabischong (1962) in the lumbricals.

Vessels of the Hand

Recently substantial information on the arterial system of the hand has been given by Coleman and Anson (1961) in a paper in which they reported on observations in 650 dissections. Throughout this paper of classic importance, due consideration is given to facts from literature. The key-stones in this literature were laid by no less than Zuckerkandl (1896), Jaschtschinski (1896) and Tandler (1896) who published their fundamental contributions in the same year, as well as in the same journal.

Zuckerkandl was primarily concerned with comparative aspects of the deep palmar arch and he found that the literature on the constitution of the deep palmar arch in man was far from conclusive. One of the major points in this regard concerns the role the ulnar artery plays in the formation of the deep palmar arch. As was already known in Zuckerkandl's days there are two routes by which the ulnar artery may anastomose with the deep palmar arch. One is through the hypothenar just along the deep branch of the ulnar nerve; the second, which has been observed in our *series no. 1899*, is between the long tendons and the hypothenar. The first-mentioned branch was called by Zuckerkandl 'ramus volaris profundus superior', the second, 'ramus volaris profundus inferior'. In the majority of his cases (74 out of 100) the two arteries occur, the inferior (distal) representing the major route. The proximal branch never failed, but the distal one was absent in 21 per cent of his cases. Zuckerkandl's comparative data will not be discussed here. It suffices to remark that the inferior branch is a typically human acquisition.

Coleman and Anson's (1961) data on the deep arch are of the same order. In 63·5 per cent of their cases two deep branches of the ulnar artery were present and again it was found that the superior ramus never failed, although in 50 per cent of the cases it does not reach so far distally as to join the deep arch. From the deep arch arise the volar metacarpal arteries. As has been observed by Fracassi (1945) in a radiological study, the metacarpal arteries usually do not extend beyond the metacarpophalangeal joint. Anastomoses with the volar digital arteries occur only in a minority of cases. Coleman and Anson found that 60 per cent of all volar metacarpal arteries do not extend further than the metacarpophalangeal joint. In 30 per cent they anastomose with the volar digital arteries. Unlike the volar digital arteries the deep volar metacarpal arteries do not relate exactly to an interspace. Instead each one relates somewhat to a metacarpal bone, although in a fairly irregular manner. The first and second volar metacarpal arteries are present in 95 per cent of their cases. Including these the smallest number found was three, the greatest six. The first volar metacarpal artery has been meticulously described by Tandler (1896) who denounced on principle its denomination as a. princeps pollicis. The a. metacarpea volaris I springs from the deep palmar arch and after a short distance passes through a slit in the adductor to reach its palmar aspect, and behind the tendon of the flexor pollicis longus it divides in two branches, a radial and an ulnar. The radial branch runs alongside the radiovolar border of the thumb, the ulnar joins the branch of the first volar common digital artery for the thumb. Tandler, dealing in much detail with the vascular supply of the thumb summarizes his findings in the following way. The ulnovolar border of the thumb is provided for by the volar common digital artery and the first volar metacarpal artery, the radiovolar border by the first volar metacarpal artery and the radial marginal artery (from the first volar digital artery); the ulnodorsal border by the first volar metacarpal artery with the first dorsal metacarpal artery and, finally, the dorsoradial border by a branch from the radial artery. The author, having established that the a. princeps pollicis is not the main artery to the thumb, strongly denounces the use of this term, concluding: 'I propose to name the art. princeps pollicis according to its position the arteria metacarpea volaris prima' (p. 279 l.c.).

It is worthwhile giving a quick glance to a few sections of *series no. 1899*, in which the a. metacarpea volaris prima is clearly visible (Fig. 3.3 and following sections). It can be seen that the artery passes between the adductor and the first metacarpal (Fig. 3.9) and then detaches a branch that passes behind the long flexor tendon, seemingly conducted by the flexor pollicis brevis. Its anastomosis with the first common digital artery, which is entirely destined for the radial side of the index, is visible in Figure 3.14, while a branch for the radial side of the thumb, visible in Figure 3.11, has been detached at levels between Figures 3.10 and 3.11. Our observations make it somewhat doubtful that this artery should pass between the two heads of the adductor as stated by Tandler. We rather believe that its course between the adductor and metacarpal I is a more natural one.

That the passage of an artery behind a tendon sheath is not uncommon can also be seen in Figure 3.11 where the fourth volar common digital artery passes behind the tendons of the little finger. This artery arises, with the ulnovolar artery of the little finger, from one common stem running outside the flexor compartment.

The pattern of vascular supply which has been confirmed by Coleman and Anson is obviously directly related to the fact that, as Coleman and Anson reported, the first volar digital artery happens to be present in 77 per cent of their material. This point in its turn is related to the formation of the superficial volar arch. It is a regular feature that the volar arch is derived entirely from the ulnar artery and has its final branch in the first volar digital artery, the latter supplying the radial side of the index and the ulnar side of the thumb. Some specification may be appropriate.

Jaschtschinski (1896) introduced a most appropriate terminology to identify the way in which the superficial volar arch is formed, a point which happens to be subject to important variation. First, two categories are distinguished, one in which an arch is formed and the other in which arch formation is absent. Jaschtschinski states that transitional forms do occur. Coleman and Anson's requirement of a complete arch (the first category), viz. that an anastomosis has to be present between the vessels that form an arch, does not seem to be applicable; the point being rather whether the vessel from which the digital volar arteries arise has an arched appearance or not. A complete arch in this sense was found by Jaschtschinski in 68 per cent of his material and by Coleman and Anson in 77 per cent of their cases. Jaschtschinski subdivided this category into four groups designated by him as (1) arcus radioulnaris, (2) arcus ulnaris, (3) arcus medianoulnaris, (4) arcus radiomedianoulnaris; a terminology which is entirely self-explanatory. The frequencies, ranked in the same order, found respectively by Jaschtschinski and by Coleman and Anson are (27; 34·5)–(38; 37)–(3; 3·8) and (—; 1·2 per cent).

The latter authors made a fifth group of those cases of ulnar arch in which an anastomosis occurs with a branch of the deep arch at the base of the thenar eminence. This type was found in 2 per cent of their cases. It is important to notice that the ulnar arch is the most frequent formation and it means that in all those cases the four interdigital arteries and the ulnar branch of the little finger arise from a superficial arch formed by the ulnar artery alone. Coleman and Anson further analyzed the patterns of the volar digital arteries and found that, disregarding the formation of the arch, in 77 per cent of these cases four common volar digital arteries are present, which means that the adjacent sides of thumb and index are supplied by branches from a common volar digital artery which, as Tandler previously observed, was the first interdigital artery. It is obvious that the distinction between the radioulnar and the ulnar arch depends on the existence of communication. In this regard it is certainly interesting to mention that Jaschtschinski found the frequency of a radioulnar arch to decrease with age and to differ in right and left hands. In his material (200) the arch was found in 27 per cent in total, right 23 per cent, left 30·9 per cent. In children (100) the total percentage was 31 per cent, in adults 23 per cent. In 20 embryos the radioulnar arch was found in eight specimens. Jaschtschinski's implicit hypothesis is obvious: that intensive use of the right hand may gradually lead to obliteration of the ramus radiopalmaris.

In each of the categories of Jaschtschinski, arch formation may gradually decrease up to complete abolition of the arch. The ulnar arch may be seen to retreat in an ulnar direction leaving the inter-digital common arteries to be supplied by the volar metacarpal arteries. This process can proceed to the ulnar branch of the fifth finger. In 12 per cent of his cases Jaschtschinski found the first common digital nerve arising from the deep arch. Coleman and Anson reported that in 13·4 per cent of their cases the first common digital artery did not arise from the superficial arch. Suppression of the radioulnar arch implies that the radiopalmar branch of the radial artery and the ulnar artery share the supply of the common digital arteries, without anastomosing.

6. CARPOMETACARPAL TRANSITION ZONE

In the area of carpometacarpal transition our main attention is focused on the first carpometacarpal joint. Haines (1944), Napier (1955a) and recently Pieron (1973) dealt with this joint both from a structural and a functional point of view. The marked convergence of ligaments towards the ulnar side of the base of the first metacarpal is a most conspicuous phenomenon. This concerns the posterior oblique ligament, the intermetacarpal ligament and the anterior oblique ligament. On the radial side the joint is bridged by one ligament only, a fairly strong one though, called the dorsoradial ligament. The significance of the position of ligaments for the well-known movement pattern of the thumb has been studied in detail by Pieron, as will be explained further in the next chapter. The mobility of the fourth and fifth carpometacarpal joints is an important feature in efficient gripping, as it facilitates to a high degree the opposition between the thumb and the two ulnar fingers.

7. THE CARPAL AREA

The discussion will be restricted to a few points only. The scaphoid tuberosity and the pisiform bone have been brought into the picture more than once, and it may be useful to mention the position of these bony structures in relation to the styloid process of both the radius and ulna. The latter processes are placed strictly on the lateral aspects of the lower arm, but the pisiform and scaphoid processes project onto the palmar aspect of the hand. This localization has some bearing on the insertion of the flexor carpi ulnaris, on the anchorage of the flexor carpi radialis and on the course of the radial artery, from the volar aspect of the radius below the long tendons of the thumb and into the 'tabatière anatomique'. We should also note that the hamulus lies distal to and slightly inward from the pisiform. This point is of importance both for the course of the inner slip of the pisometacarpal ligament (lying lateral to the hamulus and skirting its distal aspect towards the fourth metacarpal) and for the course of the deep portion of the ulnar nerve (again lying lateral to the hamulus but subsequently passing between the opponens layers towards the deep palmar space). The flexor carpi radialis tendon skirts the radial wall of the carpal tunnel as it passes towards the second and third metacarpals and so indicates the mediodistal arrangement in the anterior ligament system. This latter system is layer-wise the continuity of the anterior border of the radius and of the triangular disc: strands are added to the system from scaphoid and trapezium and from triquetrum and hamate. The system converges from both sides upon the anterior horn of the lunate; it forms a strong band in front of the capitate head and finally becomes anchored to the bases of the distal carpals. The strands mentioned above represent the most distal strands of the system.

The dorsal ligament layer is arranged quite differently: here, the prevailing direction is transverse, as is evident from the course of the radio-triquetral-scaphoid bundles.

It is rewarding to examine the positions of the dorsal tendons with respect to the radius and ulna and particularly with respect to the fibrous rings and loops that keep these tendons in position. The anchorage of these fibrous structures to bony eminences on the dorsal side of the radius (one between the extensor communis and the extensor pollicis longus, another between the latter and the dorsal wrist extensors) calls for careful attention because the loops of both the extensor communis and the extensor pollicis longus approach the bony eminence between them at an acute angle. The niches thus formed hold vascular beds for the respective tendons. It is interesting to note that the sheath of the extensor communis is rounded on its ulnar side and that of the extensor pollicis longus on its radial side. Particular attention has been paid to the position of the extensor carpi ulnaris whose tendon is held in a sheath that for all practical purposes belongs to the deep layer of the antebrachial fascia (De Leeuw, 1962; Kauer, 1968): the superficial layer of this fascia passes over the sheath and is separated from it by an areolar layer, so providing a definite degree of mobility for this sheath below the superficial fascial layer, the latter being firmly adherent to the radius.

Kauer stresses the roof tile-like arrangement of the sheaths of the extensor carpi ulnaris, the extensor digiti V and the extensor communis in the supine position of the hand. It is important to note that the sheath of the extensor carpi ulnaris, with the superficial layer firmly attached to it, becomes attached to the triangular disc, to the triquetrum and eventually incorporates the most lateral eminence of the hamate.

A point of particular importance lies in the fact that the extensor tendons bridge the proximal carpal row and also find bony support in the bases of the distal row. Earlier we described (Landsmeer, 1968) the spatial disposition of the proximal carpal row, including the specific forms of the scaphoid, of the lunate and of the capitate head. The distal carpal bones are wedge-shaped on cross-section and extend further dorsally. Being an extension of the anatomical snuffbox the subtendineal space accommodates the dorsal carpal ramifications of the radial artery; this space narrows towards the triquetrum as the radio-triquetral ligament carrying the tendon sheaths approaches this bone. The triquetral-scaphoid ligament occupies basically another layer.

The dorsal extensors of the wrist are held in a common, bilaterally rounded sheath, with the vascular bed in the middle and thus become supported by the dorsal eminence of the trapezoid, the latter projecting dorsally between these tendons. The extensor pollicis brevis and abductor pollicis longus span the entrance of the 'tabatière' to pursue their course over the first metacarpal or to become inserted into its styloid process.

A final point relates to the transformation of the fibrous loops and rings into the fascial layers which maintain the position of the tendons in the midhand. This change is a fairly simple process, but it is quite important to note that peritendineal layers reappear around the tendons, arranging themselves in such a way that the tendons become enclosed in a flat intertendineal fascia. The superficial layer of the antebrachial fascia extends over the midhand and is separated from this layer by an areolar space. In the same way an infratendineal layer comes to lie below the tendineal layer and we see that the supra- and infratendineal layers tend to fuse on the ulnar side of the fourth finger tendon and on the radial side of the index tendons. In this way a potential subfascial space is created, dorsal to the extensor communis layer. The superficial layer of the antebrachial fascia merges distally into subcutaneous layers, a process which gradually obliterates the dorsal subcutaneous space over the lower arm and wrist, and results in the subfascial space gradually becoming the subcutaneous space proper (Landsmeer, 1957). In other words the skin glides over the tendineal layer in both the distal part of the midhand and in the finger.

The tendons to the fifth finger run more or less separately in a layer below the supratendineal fascia. The tendons of the thumb also run separately from the communis complex. The supra- and infratendineal layers merge into the dorsal interosseous fascia of the first space which subsequently becomes inserted into the first metacarpal. The extensor tendons of the thumb become isolated in a fascial layer which is continuous with the fascia over the first intermetacarpal space.

8. CONCLUDING REMARKS

A study of the hand can only be sketched artificially from the vast area of comparative studies. A structural and functional study gives wide access to the fascinating comparative field throughout the animal kingdom. We have to refrain from making any attempt to discuss the abundant literature and must restrict ourselves to simply giving some access to this literature by mentioning Bishop's studies (1964) of the use of the hand in lower primates, comparative studies by Cunningham (1878), Brooks (1887), McMurrich (1903), Campbell (1939) and Lewis (1965); embryological studies by Čihák (1972), Dylevský (1972) and many others from the Prague school, who deal specifically with problems of concordance and relationships between embryological and phylogenetic patterns. Other essential works are Napier's studies (1961 and 1965) on the evolution of human grip, studies by Jouffroy and Lessertisseur (1960) on prehensile adaptations of brachiating species and more recently Tuttle's quantitative studies (1967, 1969a, 1969b and 1972) of primate hands, the latter being of unique value in the approach of relative positioning of primate species in the field of evolution.

9. Functional Considerations

1. INTRODUCTION

Because of the interdependence of function and structure it would be very artificial to report on structural aspects alone. Structural arrangement quite often directly reflects functional implications, but even in such cases the situation is generally not so simple as it may seem to be on first sight thus necessitating a more detailed analysis.

It would be beyond the scope of this treatise to survey the literature in the widest sense and in every detail. We believe that it will suffice here to elucidate the initial steps in analysis of functional order and to leave the more specialized literature to those who wish to study more deeply the analytical problems which present.

The thread of the anatomy of the hand leads us back to Albinus (1734), Camper (1760), Winslow (1752) and Weitbrecht (1742), that of its function can never bypass Duchenne (1885). The all-important point in a functional approach, and Duchenne was fully aware of it, concerns the significance of a structure in a functional pattern, e.g. it is obvious that the flexor profundus will flex the fingers and the hand, but the problem, however, is to define the role of the flexor in a well-defined pattern of flexion.

As we said above, we wish to make only some initial steps in the analysis, and so our attention is focused on the specific qualities of the individual fingers and on the significance of the position of each of the rays.

Key features of the human finger in a functional sense are the co-ordinated pattern of movement of the interphalangeal joints and the mutual independence of the metacarpophalangeal joint and the interphalangeal system. Both basic features can be tackled by the same model, the bi-muscular, bi-articular chain.

2. THE ARTICULATION OF THE FINGER

The articulation of the human finger has been approached by making use of a model system, the bi-muscular, bi-articular chain (Landsmeer, 1955, 1958, 1961). Force analysis has been carried out by Tubiana and Valentin (1963, 1964) and by Smith et al. (1964), the latter, in particular, to determine the role of finger flexors as a factor deforming the metacarpophalangeal joint in rheumatoid arthritis. Recently Fischer (1969) critically surveyed the significance, limitations and mutual interdependence of tendon displacement and force models. The model presented here is basically a tendon displacement

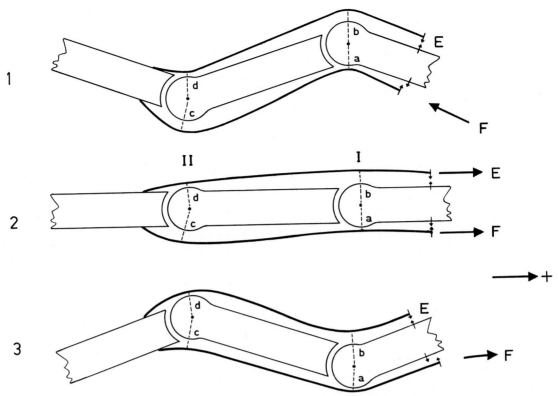

Fig. 9.1 (T 1218a; neg. 19462). A bi-muscular, bi-articular chain which explains the principle of zigzag movements; the extensor tendon is supposed to maintain its length. The flexor tendon will shorten from 2–3 and has to lengthen from 2–1.

model. It consists of two monaxial joints bridged by two antagonistic tendons. The laws, or rules, pertaining to the bi-muscular, bi-articular chain read:

(a) Given inequality in the ratios of beams of the related tendons of the two joints (Fig. 9.1), two tendons are unable to keep the system in equilibrium;

(b) the system zigzags, i.e. the intercalated bone is tilted and hence the joints begin to move in opposite directions;

(c) the direction of the zigzag in the system, or of the tilt of the intercalated bone, is determined strictly by the inequality of the relative beams. Given that a is the beam of the flexor in joint I, b is that of the extensor, c is the beam of the flexor in joint II and d is that of the extensor, then if $a/b < c/d$, the system under the influence of the two tendons will flex at joint II and extend at joint I, the flexor beam at joint II being larger, with respect to the extensor beam, than in joint I;

(d) the tilt, or zigzag, of the system will continue until in one of the joints maximum range of movement has been reached. In this particular case this will be full flexion in joint II and full extension in joint I. These positions are termed the *functional endpositions* of this system;

(e) the collapsed system, under control of the two tendons, can be moved alternate at its two joints, one of the joints being

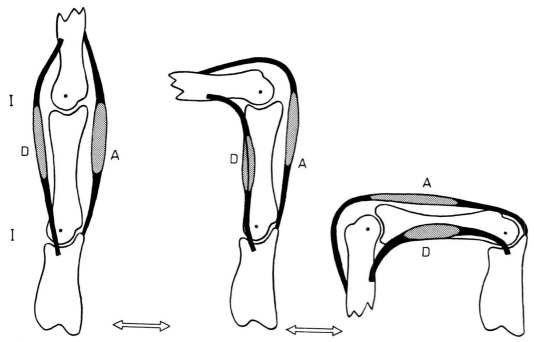

Fig. 9.2 (T. 528; neg. 7548). The alternating, or marginal movement pattern. Either of the two joints is kept in its endposition.

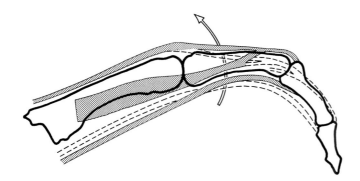

Fig. 9.3 (T 624b; neg. 10800). A third tendon, in the appropriate position, will stabilize the system. The arrow indicates the direction of tilt of the intercalated bone.

kept in functional endposition. For the system of Figure 9.2, this rule means that as long as joint I is in flexion, joint II can be flexed and extended. In turn if joint II is held extended, joint I can be flexed and extended. These alternating movements occur in the continuous sequence of curling and uncurling the system. Starting from the entirely extended position of the two joints, shortening of the flexor will flex joint I, joint II being held in extension as a result of the simultaneous action of the tendons. By means of its own tension the lengthening tendon also exerts an influence on the system. Joint I being fully flexed and hence in its functional endposition, further shortening of the flexor will lead to flexion of joint II. From full flexion of both joints, shortening of the extensor will lead first to extension of joint II and subsequently to that of joint I. It is clear that the joints cannot be moved independently of each other; hence the term *alternating movements*.

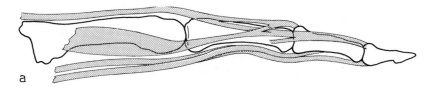

Fig. 9.4a (T. 147a; neg. 3611). Fig. 9.4b (T. 147c; neg. 3651). The tendontracks of the extensor assembly. These drawings are derived from X-rays. The various distances are therefore in accord with the real situation.

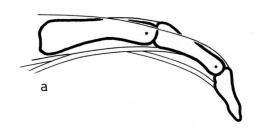

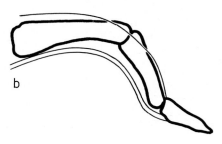

Fig. 9.5a (T. 703; neg. 10516). Fig. 9.5b (T. 703; neg. 10516). Division of the medial fascicle of the extensor assembly leads to buttonhole luxation. (a) the normal situation; (b) in absence of the median band the middle phalanx drops into ante-version.

Sometimes we term such movements 'marginal' ones. This latter term will be explained later on;

(f) the sixth rule says that a third tendon, length controlled, when added to the system and placed in appropriate position (Fig. 9.3), will render it entirely controllable, so allowing the two joints to be moved independently of each other.

a. Interphalangeal Articulation

We will apply this model first to the two interphalangeal joints, so that the middle phalanx will be considered as being the intercalated bone in a chain bridged by the extensor assembly and the flexor profundus. At this point it is logical to omit the medial band of the assembly. The middle phalanx is now bridged on its

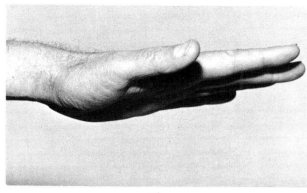

(a)

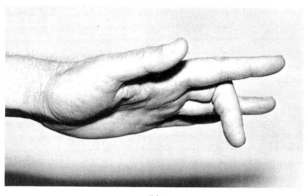

(b)

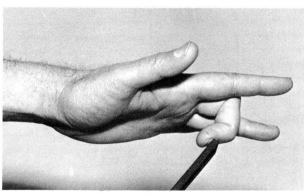

(c)

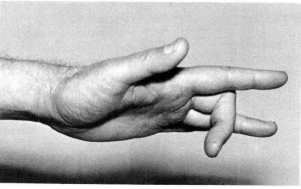

(d)

Fig. 9.6 The sequence of postures and movements which will evoke the phenomenon of release of the third phalanx and trapping of the flexor profundus tendon. 9.6a (neg. 23284):straightened fingers; 9.6b (neg. 23285):one finger flexed, which has to be done by the sublimis; 9.6c (neg. 23286):the third phalanx can only be flexed passively; 9.6d (neg. 23287):after removing the external flexor pressure, the third phalanx goes into an intermediate position; 9.6e (neg. 23288) 9.6f (neg. 23289): starting from the position of Figure 9.6a or 9.6d, the middle finger can be actively flexed by the profundus, which will, however, flex all the fingers; 9.6g (neg. 23290):extending the fingers except for the middle one. The terminal phalanx remains flexed (cf. Figs. 9.6a and 9.6d); 9.6h (neg. 23292) 9.6i (neg. 23291) 9.6j (neg. 23293):by gently pushing against its pulp, the terminal phalanx can again be released.

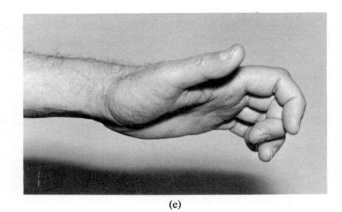

(e)

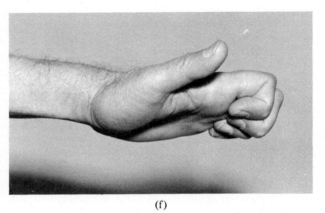

(f)

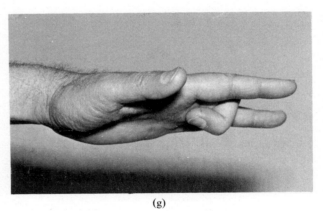

(g)

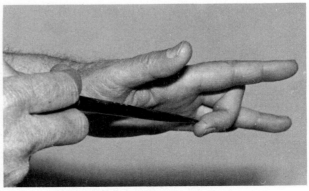

(h)

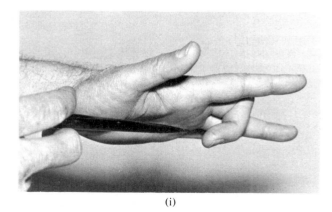

(i)

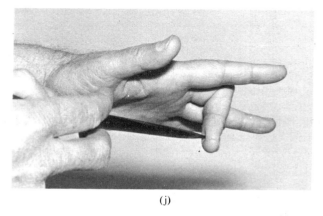

(j)

dorsal side by the lateral bands of the extensor assembly only.

Figure 9.4a and b, derived from radiographs of a finger in which
the lateral bands and the terminal tendon are wound with metal
wire, leave no doubt whatsoever that the ratio between the flexor
beam and the beam of the lateral bands of the proximal joint
considerably exceeds this same ratio in the distal joint. Hence, if
this system were to exist as such, then the middle phalanx subjected
to the influence of the extensor and the flexor profundus simultaneously
would make a forward tilt; flexing at the proximal interphalangeal
joint and extending at the distal interphalangeal one. This collapse
of the system leads to a position well known from pathology, viz.
the *déformité de boutonnière* or the buttonhole luxation (Fig. 9.5b).
It should be stressed that this collapse will inevitably occur in the
absence of the medial band, which means that in those cases in
which trauma has divided the medial band only, the buttonhole
deformity shows virtually the *normal disposition of the middle phalanx*.
Put alternately, the middle phalanx in the chain of the finger is
continuously subjected to an influence of anteversion. The actual
anteversion is normally arrested by the medial band of the extensor
assembly (Fig. 9.5a). The flexor sublimis, in principle, reinforces
the anteversion. The result is obvious: the middle phalanx continuously loads the medial band of the extensor assembly. This
conclusion can be extended logically by the concept that both the
second and third phalanges are suspended from offshoots of the
extensor assembly, the middle phalanx being suspended from the

medial band of the extensor assembly and the terminal phalanx from the terminal tendon of this system.

We have now to look more closely at the problem embodied in the fact that during flexion both interphalangeal joints show a co-ordinated pattern, as they do also during extension. A functional phenomenon which can be seen as a key to the co-ordination pattern is the so-called phenomenon of the loosened third phalanx, which can be easily evoked in the living hand in the following way (Figs. 9.6a–j).

First extend all fingers at metacarpophalangeal and interphalangeal joints (Fig. 9.6a). Then flex one of the fingers at the proximal interphalangeal joint, keeping the others firmly extended (Fig. 9.6b). In this position the terminal phalanx of the finger flexed at the proximal interphalangeal joint is quite beyond voluntary control. By gently pushing its nail this phalanx can readily be made to flex (Fig. 9.6c), and on removal of this force it tends to spring back, although not into the fully extended position (Fig. 9.6d). Full extension can be achieved only passively, by gently pushing against the pulp surface. The position in Figure 9.6b represents the initial phase of a quite intriguing phenomenon, viz. the trapping of the deep flexor tendon. Contraction of the flexor profundus will flex the third phalanx; this contraction can be evoked by starting flexion of the terminal phalanges of the fingers held extended as in Figure 9.6e. We can now see the gradual flexion of the released phalanx, a flexion that can in no way be counteracted by the extensor communis. All phalanges being flexed (Fig. 9.6f), it may now again be attempted to evoke the release of the third phalanx of one finger by extending the others, but with some surprise we find that the third phalanx of the non-extending finger remains flexed (Fig. 9.6g). It turns out, however, that it is not the contraction of the profundus that keeps the phalanx flexed, because the phalanx can be easily released from this flexed position by gentle external force (Fig. 9.6h, i, j). Now again the third phalanx is in the loosened or released condition. The explanation of this phenomenon is quite simple, in that the flexor profundus tendon becomes trapped in the chiasma tendineum of the superficial flexor during its proximal shift. This entrapment is more effective with concomitant contraction of the flexor sublimis. It is obvious that it requires hardly any force at all to pull the tendon distally through this trap, the flexor profundus again being released.

The phenomenon of the loosened third phalanx is based on the position of the bands, or tendons, of the extensor assembly at the proximal interphalangeal joint. Cross-sections at the level of the trochlea of the first phalanx are extremely instructive. The two lateral bands situated on the shoulders of the trochlea lie nearer the axis of rotation of the proximal interphalangeal joint than the median band, which runs over the dorsum of the trochlea. This situation implies that to allow flexion of the joint less length is needed for the lateral bands than for the medial band. However, as a result of the presence of an extensor assembly, a distal pull on either the medial band or on the lateral bands will make the whole assembly shift distally over the dorsum of the first phalanx. Hence flexion of the middle phalanx entails a certain distal shift of the extensor

indicate the distribution of phalangeal tendons and their relation
to spherical and cylindrical grips (Landsmeer, 1955) (Figs. 9.13a
b, c, d).

Differentiation of function within one interosseus could not be
detected by the electromyograph.

Another point is the synergic interaction between the two interossei
of each finger, which is seen quite regularly in those resisted movements of the hands, as in gripping when two interossei are active.
This is particularly noticeable in the index, but is also seen in the
little and ring fingers.

Interesting data on intrinsic activity were collected during 'precision handling'. Meibuhr investigated as many as eight movements,
each of them during handling and on return to rest. In the handling
phase the fingers are in contact with a tracking device which provides
some resistance to the motion. The return phase is entirely unloaded,
the fingers having no contact with each other.

Precision acts, such as pad-to-pad and tip-to-tip rotation, show
precisely the role of interossei in positioning the finger. In clockwise
rotation between thumb and index, palmar II (I) is highly active and
in anticlockwise rotation dorsal I starts firing and palmar II stops.
It should be noted that this pattern applies in both loaded and
unloaded condition, i.e. either with the fingers actually in contact
with each other or just sliding over each other. The activity of the
so-called 'thenar triad', the opponens pollicis, the abductor pollicis
brevis and the flexor is quite conspicuous in these various motion
patterns. In the return phase of clockwise rotation and in the
handling phase of anticlockwise rotation, both tip-to-tip and pad-to-
pad, the thenar triad is found to be extremely active; this is also seen
in a translation movement 'away from the palm' in the loaded
condition, while in the unloaded condition the flexor pollicis brevis
drops out from the triad. In the motion toward the palm the triad
is active only in the loaded condition. The unloaded motion toward
the palm (or return phase of the motion away from the palm) is
a purely extrinsic affair and the intrinsics are entirely silent. This is
quite interesting because it means that this motion is virtually a true
clawing motion. The movement towards the palm with the fingers
in contact with an object immediately evokes activity of the thenar
triad and of both interossei.

These findings can be summarized in this way that in writing
both the upstroke and the downstroke involves the intrinsics except
that during the downstroke (motion toward the palm), the lumbrical
drops out. The activity of the lumbrical in the loaded movement away
from the palm seems to tally well with its role in interphalangeal
extension and lumbrical silence in both movements towards the palm,
both loaded and unloaded, does not seem too surprising. Interphalangeal flexion never evokes lumbrical activity.

In this context, it is very interesting to observe lumbrical activity
in the gentle pinch, both pad-to-pad and tip-to-tip. Again all
intrinsics, the abductor pollicis brevis minimally, but the adductor
significantly, are active, including the lumbrical. The interesting and
intriguing point is that if pinch becomes a movement towards the
palm, loaded or unloaded, the lumbrical stops acting. These data
on lumbrical activity are quite consistent with those reported on

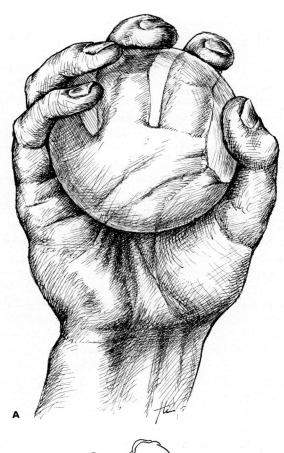

Fig. 9.13a (T. 101; neg. 3032).

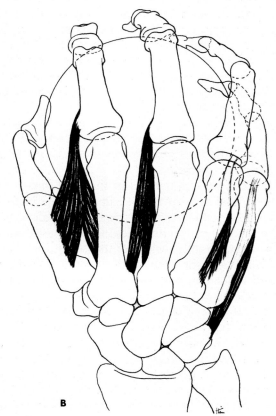

Fig. 9.13b (T. 107; neg. 3312).

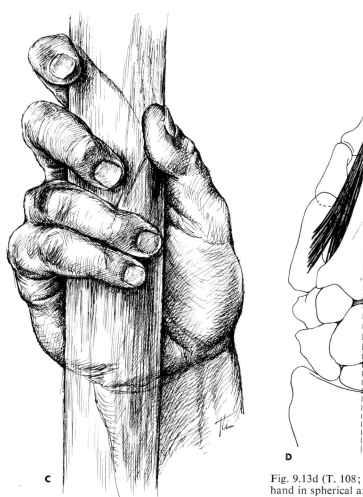

C

Fig. 9.13c (T. 102; neg. 3033).

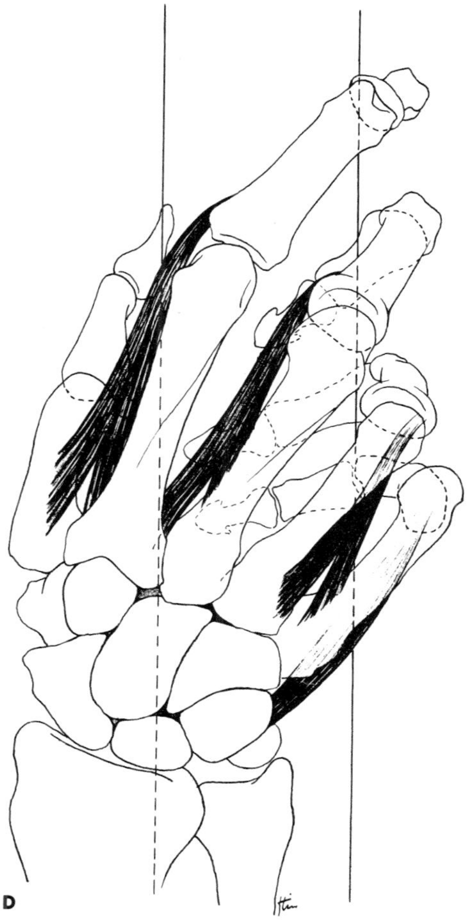

D

Fig. 9.13d (T. 108; neg. 3313). Drawings of a hand in spherical and in cylindrical grip positions. In drawings of X-rays of these postures, those interossei with a phalangeal insertion (a–d) have been pictured.

free movement of the hand. Again, the lumbrical comes into play as soon as interphalangeal extension is required or interphalangeal flexion has to be avoided, as in pinching.

As for the shaping of the hand to produce an efficient grip, we have already referred to the asymmetry of the metacarpophalangeal joints which is reflected in the asymmetry of the head of each metacarpal; the asymmetry in size and position of the metacarpophalangeal ligaments; the asymmetrical disposition of the phalangeal base and we have also mentioned the asymmetrical position of the head with respect to the axes of the corresponding metacarpal, in the index, the ring and little fingers (Chapter 8).

6. THUMB ARTICULATION

Literature on the thumb has been surveyed in a brilliant and thorough way by Ebskov (1970) who also made a substantial contribution to the functional analysis of extrinsic and intrinsic thumb musculature, using electromyography. To the time of writing designation and terminology of thumb movements have not been resolved satisfactorily and the existing confusion calls for an elementary *de novo* approach. It is not surprising that Ebskov did not opt for one of the terminologies coined in the literature, but chose to mark the position of the thumb, with respect to the plane of the hand, on those circles through which the thumb is supposed to pass during extreme circumduction and during a similar motion when the thumb remains as close to the hand as possible.

Movements of the thumb from the outer arch towards the hand are all termed 'adduction' and in the reverse direction, they are all termed 'abduction'; all such latter movements place the thumb somewhere on the circumduction curve.

In this concept it is obviously necessary to make a few specifications and to distinguish volar abduction from radial abduction. This terminological model should be basically restricted to indicate those movements which are produced in the carpometacarpal joint. In fact, de la Caffinière (1970) in his approach of the displacements of the first metacarpal distinguished 'la grande et la petite course du premier métacarpien' and later Pieron (1973) followed the same trend where he distinguished the radial and the ulnar curves on the path described by the head of the first metacarpal. Both de la Caffinière and Pieron strictly related this pathway to the plane of the dorsum of the second and third metacarpals, as a metacarpal plane as such cannot have been unequivocally determined.

Movements of the metacarpophalangeal and the interphalangeal joint should be superimposed in the metacarpal cone, which is a complicated procedure. Alternately it should not be forgotten that a term such as 'opposition' indicates a movement resulting from a most complex articular mechanism. Virtually, this movement involves three joints of the thumb, the chains of the fingers involved and, when the fourth and fifth fingers participate, the carpometacarpal joints of the fingers concerned. In this respect it is important to realize that the first metacarpal head, even in extreme opposition, does not project over the second metacarpal as long as the plane of the dorsum of the second and third metacarpals is taken as the plane of projection.

Studies by Haines (1944), Napier (1955a), de la Caffinière (1970) and Pieron (1973) on the ligament apparatus have enabled us to distinguish four ligaments of the carpometacarpal joint, viz. the posterior oblique and intermetacarpal ligaments converging on the volar-ulnar tubercle of metacarpal I (Figs. 9.14a and b) the anterior oblique ligament running an oblique course and being inserted into the volar aspect of metacarpal I and finally a radially placed ligament, termed by de la Caffinière 'le ligament droit antéro-externe' and by Pieron the 'dorso-radial ligament'.

The role of the ligaments in producing axial rotation is now fully recognized. Pronation along the radial curve (la grande course) and supination along the ulnar curvature (la petite course) are seen in Figures 9.15a and b from Pieron, who made a detailed analysis of the displacement of joint contact throughout circumduction. In these same figures the results of his analysis can be easily read. The asymmetrical form of the circumduction curve reflects the asymmetry of the joint surface of the trapezium. Axial rotation cannot be

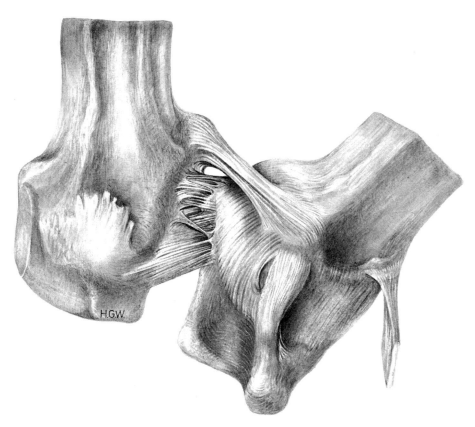

Fig. 9.14a (T. 1649; neg. 23900).

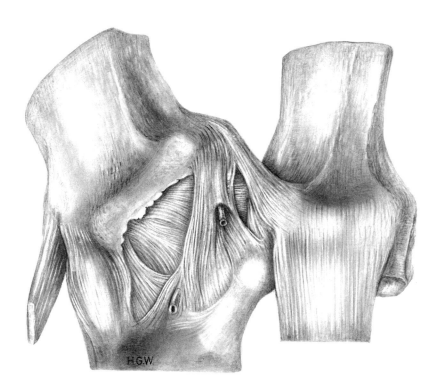

Fig. 9.14b (T. 1648; neg. 23901).
Drawings of the ligaments of the
carpometacarpal joint of the thumb.
(a) anterior view; (b) view from the posterior and distal side (from Pieron, 1973).

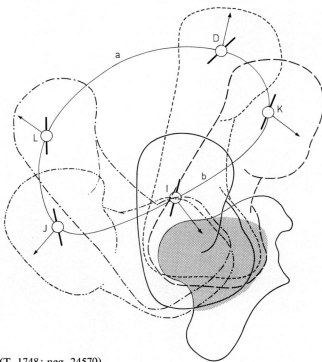

Fig. 9.15a (T. 1748; neg. 24570).

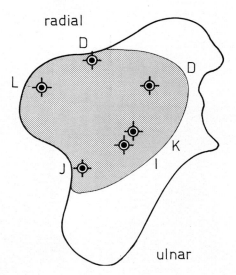

Fig. 9.15b (T. 1779a; neg. 24997). (a) drawing of superimposed X-rays taken in a disto-proximal direction of metacarpal I and trapezium. (a) the radial curve, (b) the ulnar curve. The arrows indicate the direction of traction. The rotation is indicated by the short lines; (b) The areas of contact on the trapezium in the corresponding positions of metacarpal I (from Pieron, 1973).

performed as an independent motion primarily because the irregular shape of the articular surfaces precludes such a motion (Kuczynski, 1974), and secondly because the muscular system is not equipped with a sufficient number of muscles to carry out such a movement.

Electromyography of both the thenar and extrinsic thumb muscles has been carried out by Ebskov (1970) and by Hamonet *et al.* (1972). To relate these data to the movements of the thumb Ebskov and Boe (1968) made use of 'the hexatron', a goniometer designed by these authors. The thumb was attached to the apparatus by means of a splint which immobilized the interphalangeal joint. It was assumed

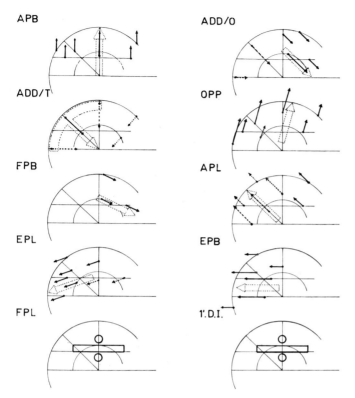

Fig. 9.16 *Spectrum of Activity: Muscle by Muscle.* The diagrams illustrate the functions of ten thumb muscles in cyclic, unloaded motion of the finger, and represent the functional conclusions, based on the present investigation.

The arrows designate the probable importance of the muscle in the various test motions. ⟶: particular importance; – – – ⟶: probable, possibly particular importance; ⟶: probable importance; – – ⟶: dubious importance; ▭⟩: probable prime function of the muscle. (From Ebskov, 1970)

that what Ebskov termed 'total thumb movement' could be represented by the polar co-ordinates of the splinted phalanges. These polar co-ordinates were subsequently used to determine the path of the thumb which in turn made it possible to process data statistically.

Eventually Ebskov put forward his results in a 'tendency concept' meaning that the probable importance of a muscle in a given movement could be described as being of 'particular importance', 'probable possible importance', 'probable importance' and 'dubious importance', the resultant giving a probable prime function of the muscle. In this way a spectrum of activities could be established for each movement, muscle by muscle. The latter spectrum, pictured in Figure 9.16, summarizes these results in a most surveyable manner.

It is of some importance to note that Ebskov took the course of the tip of the thumb as being representative of what he called 'total thumb motion'. Hamonet *et al.* registered the course of the head of the first metacarpal instead and they related the activity of various thenar muscles to the location of the curve or the radius along which the motion was taking place. Working along these lines Hamonet *et al.* summarized the activity pattern of the thenar muscles as follows.

The adductor appears to be active in all motions in which the first metacarpal approaches the second, no matter where the point of departure.

The short abductor shows activity during opposition (the greater course) and in all motions in which the first metacarpal moves away from the second metacarpal.

The opponens pollicis is active during opposition and, to some extent, during abduction, while the short flexor appears to be primarily an opposing muscle.

Though we do not want to detract from the importance of E.M.G. data, these data alone do not tell us about such things as the conditions of equilibrium and of stability in the articular system of the thumb. The effect of the extrinsic muscles of the thumb will be reflected in its position during clinical intrinsic paralysis and it is true that pinching with arched fingers and thumb becomes impossible when only residual pinch remains, which is known as Froment's sign. Hence the strut of the first metacarpal cannot be set out, a mechanism which obviously requires the activity of the intrinsic muscles, while as for the activity pattern of these muscles, it is not too surprising to find that it depends largely on the direction of the opposition as to which muscle or muscles become active.

However, we should not overlook the fact that while most of the thenar muscles, including the adductor, are inserted into the sesamoids and the base of the first phalanx, only one, the opponens, is inserted into the first metacarpal, which also receives the abductor longus. It is obvious that an analytical model of the thumb which will explain the mutual relations of the thenar muscles is badly needed. In designing such a model, due consideration should be given to the mechanical interactions between the muscular system and the ligaments of the carpometacarpal joint.

7. CARPAL FUNCTION

Recent advances made in the approach of carpal mechanism (Van Lamoen in Matricali, 1961; Kauer, 1964, 1974 and Mulder, 1970) tend to isolate the following features as being of great relevance in a functional respect.

(1) The presence of longitudinal articulation chains, the radius-scaphoid-trapezoid chain and the radius-lunate-capitate chain;

(2) the linkage of these two chains, by the capitate which articulates with the scaphoid as well the lunate and by the ligament between lunate and scaphoid. It is important to observe that the head of the capitate is provided with articular facets which are differently curved and, further, that on the distal surface of the radius two facets can be distinguished, one for the scaphoid and one for the lunate, which are separated by a crest.

Several conclusions related to the functional mechanism of this arrangement are permissible.

The scaphoid and lunate cannot articulate as an immobile block with the radius, at least not during abduction and Kauer (1964, 1974) showed that owing to the differences in curvature between scaphoid and lunate this is also true during flexion. Even if the articulation mechanism consisting of scaphoid, lunate and capitate head were to exist on its own, it would be impossible for the scaphoid to articulate in a fossa of rigid form. In fact, a cross-section such as that in Figure 2.5 shows clearly that articulation of the capitate

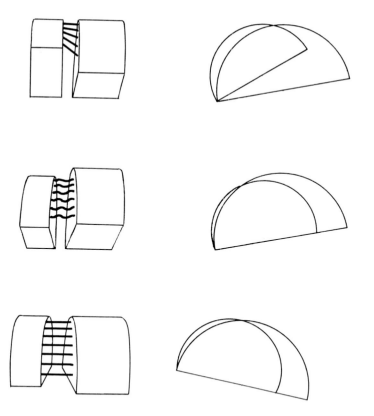

Fig. 9.17 (T. 919; neg. 14384).
Diagrammatic model to explain the mode
of movement of eccentric bodies, which
move around a common axis at one side
while at the other side they are allowed
limited motion. In the middle drawings
the smaller body looses contact with a
horizontal plane. In the lower drawings
the contact is re-established while the
bodies have approached each other
(from Kauer, 1964).

head in the socket formed by scaphoid and lunate will lead directly
to a mutual displacement of the scaphoid and lunate.

The fact that the lunate and scaphoid act as intercalated bones
means that, because of their wedge shape, they tend to escape from
the chain in an anterior direction, the lunate being arrested by the
anterior ligament layer, and the scaphoid by butting against the
trapezium and trapezoid.

Any movement of the distal row, and so of the hand, will be
conveyed to the proximal row, but as we have observed, it is impossible for the proximal row to articulate with the radius without
the mutual displacement of the lunate and scaphoid. The continuous
adjustment of the proximal row is controlled by a remarkable combined action of the interosseous ligament between scaphoid and lunate,
the irregular form of the scaphoid head and the facet on the capitate
head. As has been shown by Kauer (1964 and 1974) the anterior
fibres of the interosseous ligament are longer than the posterior
ones. At the posterior end the scaphoid and lunate have a centre of
movement, while at the anterior end the interosseous ligament allows
scaphoid and lunate some mutual displacement, either as a proximo-
distal shift or as a movement away from each other, so that a
small gap opens between the two bones. These movements take place
around a centre located posteriorly, where the fibres of the interosseous ligament are much shorter than anteriorly (Fig. 9.17).

It is important to recognize that both scaphoid and lunate are
able to make a swerving movement around the capitate head,
guided by its two facets. During flexion scaphoid and lunate move
not only in a sagittal plane and in abduction not only in frontal

and sagittal planes. Both scaphoid and lunate are subjected to small longitudinal rotations. The interplay between distal and proximal rows produces an action between scaphoid and lunate which ensures a continuous adaption of the proximal row to the distal one and to the radius. This mechanism gives the carpus great stability. The parallel chains are linked to each other and freely permit flexion, abduction and all combined movements such as circumduction, but rigorously exclude rotation. The latter quality is a prerequisite for the proper functioning of pronation and supination. As the latter movement has to be conveyed from the forearm to the hand, freedom of rotation would immediately jeopardize this essential function of the human hand.

The role played by the triquetrum in carpal function is still somewhat enigmatic, but the bone seemingly must play a conspicuous role in the ligamentous control of carpal function. As we saw in Chapter II the triquetrum represents a stronghold of attachment for both dorsal (radiocarpal and the ligament from triquetrum to scaphoid) and volar ligaments (the triquetrum-lunate interosseal linkage and the triquetrum-capitate, triquetrum-hamate connections). In this regard full attention should be given to fibres from the interarticular disc, being attached to the triquetrum (Kauer, 1964 and 1974). The interposition of a fibrous pad between styloid process and triquetrum was considered by Lewis (1965b, 1969 and 1970) in the context of the phylogenetic development of pronation and supination.

We have not included a survey of the musculature of the lower arm because it would have taken us too far from the area of our particular study. Referring to studies of Fahrer (1969) it is readily apparent that an important aspect of the function of the hand lies in the structure of the extrinsic muscles of the fingers. Restrictions imposed upon the fingers related to their independent function are seen in the juncturae tendineae on the dorsal side of the metacarpus and the separation of the flexor tendons, or in both, and any diagnostic procedure should be able to discriminate between these structural arrangements. Recently Shrewsbury and Kuczynski (1974) made a detailed study of the chiasma of the flexor digitorum sublimis.

We have deliberately left out directions for clinical investigation because this is clearly beyond our competence. There are also many other points that have not been covered, such as dermatoglyphs, metrical data, anthropological and developmental aspects, including congenital malformations, to mention but a few of them.

We feel that such an extension would conflict with our primary aim of producing an atlas of the hand and of projecting our findings against a background of general information.

Bibliography

ALBINUS, B. S. (1734) *Historia Musculorum Hominis*, pp. 508–513. Leiden.

ANDERSON, W. (1894) A note on the course and relations of the deep branch of the ulnar nerve. *Journal of Anatomy and Physiology*, **28**, x–xii.

ANSON, B. J. (1963) *An Atlas of Human Anatomy*. 2nd edn. Philadelphia: Saunders.

ANSON, B. J. & ASHLEY, F. L. (1940) The midpalmar compartment, associated spaces and limiting layers. *Anatomical Record*, **78**, 389–408.

BACKHOUSE, K. M. & CATTON, W. T. (1954) An experimental study of the functions of the lumbrical muscles in the human hand. *Journal of Anatomy*, **88**, 133–141.

BISHOP, ALISON (1964) Use of the hand in lower primates. In *Evolutionary and Genetic Biology of Primates*, ed. Buettner-Janusch, J., pp. 133–225. New York: Academic Press.

BOJSEN-MØLLER, F. & SCHMIDT, L. (1974) The palmar aponeurosis and the central spaces of the hand. *Journal of Anatomy*, **117**, 55–68.

BROOKS, H. ST. J. (1886) Variations in the nerve supply of the flexor brevis pollicis muscle. *Journal of Anatomy and Physiology*, **20**, 641–644.

BROOKS, H. ST. J. (1887) On the short muscles of the pollex and hallux of the anthropoid apes, with special reference to the opponens hallucis. *Journal of Anatomy*, **22**, 78–95.

BROOKS, H. ST. J. (1888) On the distribution of the cutaneous nerves on the dorsum of the human hand. *Transactions of the Royal Academy of Medicine of Ireland*, **6**, 463–472.

CAFFINIÈRE, J.-Y. DE LA (1970) L'articulation trapézo-métacarpienne approche bio-mécanique et appareil ligamentaire. *Archives d'Anatomie Pathologique*, **18**, 277–284.

CAMPBELL, B. (1939) The comparative anatomy of the dorsal interosseous muscles. *Anatomical Record*, **73**, 115–125.

CAMPER, P. (1760) *Demonstrationum anatomico-pathologicarum*. Liber primus. *Continens brachii humani fabricum et morbos*. Amsterdam.

CANNIEU, A. (1897) Note sur une anastomose entre la branche profonde du cubital et le médian. *Bulletin de la Société d'Anatomie de Bordeaux*, **18**, 339–340.

ČIHÁK, R. (1972) Ontogenesis of the skeleton and intrinsic muscles of the human hand and foot. *Ergebnisse der Anatomie und Entwicklungsgeschichte*, **46**, 1–194.

CLELAND, R. (1878) On the cutaneous ligaments of the phalanges. *Journal of Anatomy and Physiology*, **12**, 526–527.

COLEMAN, S. S. & ANSON, B. J. (1961) Arterial patterns in the hand based upon a study of 650 specimens. *Surgery, Gynecology and Obstetrics*, **113**, 408–424.

CRUVEILHIER, J. (1843) *Traité d'Anatomie Descriptive*. 2nd edn. Paris: Labe.

CUNNINGHAM, J. (1878) The intrinsic muscles of the hand of the Thylacine (Thylacinus Cynocephalus), Cuscus (Phalangista Maculata), and Phascogale (Phascogale Calura). *Journal of Anatomy and Physiology*, **12**, 434–444.

DAY, M. H. & NAPIER, J. R. (1961) The two heads of flexor pollicis brevis. *Journal of Anatomy*, **95**, 123–130.

DUCHENNE, G. B. (1885) *Physiologie der Bewegungen nach elektrischen Versuchen und klinischen Beobachtungen mit Anwendungen auf das Studium der Lähmungen und Entstellungen*. (Aus dem Französischen übersetzt von Dr. C. Wernicke.) Cassel und Berlin: Theodor Fischer.

DYLEVSKÝ, I. (1972) Cited in article by Čihák, R., in *Ergebdisse der Anatomie und Entwicklungsgeschichte*, **46**, 180.

EBSKOV, B. (1970) De motibus motoribusque pollicis humani. Thesis: Copenhagen, Denmark.

EBSKOV, B. & BOE, C. (1966) The Hexatron, a new thumb goniometer. *Acta Orthopaedica Scandinavica*, **37**, 58–66.

FAHRER, M. (1969) The range of movement of the fourth metacarpal joint: a problem for pianists and anatomists. *Journal of Anatomy*, **104**, 410.

FERRARINI, M. (1936) Morfogenesi della aponevrosi palmare. *Archivo Italiano di Anatomia e di Embryologia*, **37**, 203–268.

FISCHER, G. W. (1969) A treatise on the topographical anatomy of the long finger and a biomechanical investigation of its interjoint movement. Thesis: University of Iowa, USA.

FORREST, W. J. (1967) Motor innervation of human thenar and hypothenar muscles in 25 hands: a study combining E.M.G. and percutaneous nerve stimulation. *Canadian Journal of Surgery*, **10**, 196–199.

FRACASSI, H. (1945) Arterias interosseas de la mano. *Prensa Medica Argentina* (Buenos Aires), **32**, 27–30.

FROHSE, F. (1906) Die Aponeurosis palmaris und digitalis der menschlichen Hand mit besonderer Berücksichtigung ihrer Funktion. *Archiv für Anatomie und Physiologie. Anat. Abt. Archiv für Anatomie und Entwicklungsgeschichte*, pp. 101–108.

GAUL, J. ST. (1971) The ratio of motion of the interphalangeal joints. (Unpublished report.)

GEHWOLF, SOPHIE VON (1921) Plexusbildung in der Hohlhand. *Anatomischer Anzeiger*, **54**, 435–440.

GRAY, D. J. & GARDNER, E. (1965) The innervation of the joints of the wrist and hand. *Anatomical Record*, **151**, 261–266.

GRODINSKY, M. & HOLYOKE, A. (1941) The fasciae and fascial spaces of the palm. *Anatomical Record*, **79**, 435–451.

HAINES, W. H. (1944) The mechanism of rotation at the first carpometacarpal joint. *Journal of Anatomy*, **78**, 44–46.

HAINES, W. H. (1951) The extensor apparatus of the finger. *Journal of Anatomy*, **85**, 251–259.

HALL, ELISABETH A. (1968) Electromyography of the intrinsic hand muscles in power grip. Thesis: Case Western Reserve University, Cleveland, Ohio, USA.

HAMONET, C., CAFFINIÈRE, J.-Y. DE LA & OPSOMER, G. (1972) Mouvements du pouce: détermination électro-myographique des secteurs d'activité des muscles thénariens. *Archives d'Anatomie Pathologique*, **20**, 363–367.

HARNESS, D. & SEKELES, E. (1971) The double anastomotic innervation of thenar muscles. *Journal of Anatomy*, **109**, 461–466.

HARNESS, D., SEKELES, E. & CHACO, J. (1974) The double motor innervation of the opponens pollicis muscles: an electromyographic study. *Journal of Anatomy*, **117**, 239–331.

HARTMANN, H. (1887) Note sur l'anatomie des nerfs de la paume de la main. *Bulletins de la Société Anatomique de Paris*, pp. 860–864.

HAUCK, G. (1923) Die Ruptur der Dorsalaponeurose am ersten Interphalangealgelenk, zugleich ein Beitrag zur Anatomie und Physiologie der Dorsalaponeurose. *Archiv für klinische Chirurgie*, **123**, 197–232.

HÉDON. (1889) Étude critique sur l'innervation de la face dorsale de la main. *Journal International d'Anatomie et de Physiologie*, **6**, 141–158.

HOLCOMB, G. R., IRVING, T. E. & SMITH, R. D. (1958) Coronal deviation and tilt in the proximal interphalangeal joints of man. *American Journal of Physical Anthropology*, **16**, 429–440.

HOVELACQUE, A. (1927) *Anatomie des Nerfs Craniens et Rachidiens et du Système Grand Sympathique Chez L'homme.* Paris: Gaston Doin.

JASCHTSCHINSKI, S. N. (1896) Morphologie und Topographie des Arcus Volaris Sublimis und Profundus. *Anatomische Hefte*, Abt. I, **7**, 163–188.

JOUFFROY, F. K. & LESSERTISSEUR, J. (1960) Les spécialisations anatomiques de la main chez les singes à progression suspendue. *Mammalia*, **24**, 93–151.

KANAVEL, A. B. (1925) *Infections of the Hand.* 5th edn. Philadelphia: Lea & Febiger.

KAPLAN, E. B. (1966) *Functional and Surgical Anatomy of the Hand.* 2nd edn. Philadelphia: Lippincott.

KAUER, J. M. G. (1964) Een analyse van de carpale flexie. Thesis: Leiden, Holland.

KAUER, J. M. G. (1968) L'extension du ligament triangulaire dans la région carpienne. *Comptes Rendus de l'Association des Anatomistes*, **142**, 1048–1056.

KAUER, J. M. G. (1974) The interdependence of carpal articulation chains. *Acta anatomica*, **88**, 481–501.

KIRK, T. S. (1924) Some points in the mechanism of the human hand. *Journal of Anatomy*, **58**, 228–230.

KUCZYNSKI, K. (1968) The proximal interphalangeal joint. *Journal of Bone and Joint Surgery*, **50-B**, 656–663.

KUCZYNSKI, K. (1974) Carpometacarpal joint of the human thumb. *Journal of Anatomy*, **118**, 119–126.

LAMOEN IN MATRICALI, E. A. M. VAN. (1961) Ontleedkundig-functioneel onderzoek van het polsgewricht. Thesis: Leiden, Holland.

LANDSMEER, J. M. F. (1949) The anatomy of the dorsal aponeurosis of the human finger and its functional significance. *Anatomical Record*, **104**, 31–44.

LANDSMEER, J. M. F. (1955) Anatomical and functional investigations on the articulation of the human fingers. *Acta anatomica*, Suppl. 24, **25**, 1–69.

LANDSMEER, J. M. F. (1957) Les aponévroses dorsales de la main. *Comptes Rendus de l'Association des Anatomistes*, **95**, 443–449.

LANDSMEER, J. M. F. (1958) A report on the co-ordination of the interphalangeal joints of the human finger and its disturbances. *Acta Morphologica Neerlando-Scandinavica*, **2**, 59–84.

LANDSMEER, J. M. F. (1961) Studies in the anatomy of articulation. I. The equilibrium of the 'intercalated' bone. *Acta Morphologica Neerlando-Scandinavica*, **3**, 287–303. II. Patterns of movement of bi-muscular, bi-articular systems. *Acta Morphologica Neerlando-Scandinavica*, **3**, 304–321.

LANDSMEER, J. M. F. (1962) Power grip and precision handling. *Annals of the Rheumatic Diseases*, **21**, 164–170.

LANDSMEER, J. M. F. (1965) Structural analysis of the fourth dorsal interosseus of the human hand. *Acta anatomica*, **62**, 176–214.

LANDSMEER, J. M. F. (1966) Analyse de la structure des interosseux dorsaux II et III. *Comptes Rendus de l'Association des Anatomistes*, **132**, 590–595.

LANDSMEER, J. M. F. (1968) Les cohérences spatiales et l'équilibre spatial dans la région carpienne. *Acta anatomica*, Suppl. 54, **70**, 1–84.

LANDSMEER, J. M. F. (1972) Some observations on the extensor assembly in Saimiri sciurea. *Journal of Anatomy*, **113**, 276.

LANDSMEER, J. M. F. (1973) The extensor assembly of Saimiri sciurea. *Folia Morphologica*, **21**, 209–211.

LANDSMEER, J. M. F. (1974) The extensor assembly in some primate species (in preparation).

LANDSMEER, J. M. F. & ANSINGH, H. R. (1957) X-ray observations on rotation of the fingers in the metacarpophalangeal joints. *Acta anatomica*, **30**, 404–410.

LANDSMEER, J. M. F. & LONG, C. (1965) The mechanism of finger control, based on electromyograms and location analysis. *Acta anatomica*, **60**, 330–347.

LEEUW, B. DE (1962) De stratigrafie van het dorsale polsgebied als uitgangspunt voor een onderzoek naar de positie van de m. extensor carpi ulnaris tijdens het proneren en supineren van de onderarm. Thesis: Leiden, Holland.

LEGUEU, F. & JUVARA, E. (1892) Des aponévroses de la paume de la main. *Bulletins de la Société Anatomique de Paris*, **67**, 383–400.

LEWIS, O. J. (1965a) The evolution of the Mm. Interossei in the primate hand. *Anatomical Record*, **153**, 275–288.

LEWIS, O. J. (1965b) Evolutionary change in the primate wrist and inferior radio-ulnar joints. *Anatomical Record*, **151**, 275–286.

LEWIS, O. J. (1969) The Hominoid wrist joint. *American Journal of Physical Anthropology*, **30**, 251–268.

LEWIS, O. J., HAMSHERE, R. J. & BUCKNILL, T. M. (1970) The anatomy of the wrist joint. *Journal of Anatomy*, **106**, 539–552.

LONG, C. (1970) *Normal and Abnormal Motor Control in the Upper Extremities*. Final Report. Social and Rehabilitation Services. Grant No. RD-2377-M. Dec. 1966 to April 1970.

LONG, C. & BROWN, MARY E. (1964) Electromyographic kinesiology of the hand: muscles moving the long finger. *Journal of Bone and Joint Surgery*, **46-A**, 1683–1706.

MANNERFELT, L. (1964) Studies on an anastomosis between the median and ulnar nerves in the forearm. *Acta Universitatis Lundensis*, Section II, no. 6.

MANNERFELT, L. (1966) Studies on the hand in ulnar nerve paralysis. A clinical experimental investigation in normal and anomalous innervation. *Acta Orthopaedica Scandinavica*, Suppl. 87.

MASLIEURAT-LAGÉMARD, G. E. (1839) De l'anatomie descriptive et chirurgicale des aponévroses et des membranes synoviales de la main, de leur application à la thérapeutique et à la médecine opératoire. *Gazette Médicale de Paris*, **7**, 273–280.

MCMURRICH, J. P. (1903) The phylogeny of the forearm flexors. *American Journal of Anatomy*, **2**, 177–209.

MEIBUHR, SUSAN L. (1969) Electromyography of intrinsic muscles of the hand during precision handling. Thesis: Case Western Reserve University, Cleveland, Ohio, USA.

MILLER, M. R., RALSTON, H. J. & KASAHARA, M. (1958) The pattern of cutaneous innervation of the human hand. *American Journal of Anatomy*, **102**, 183–218.

MONTANT, R. & BAUMANN, A. (1937) Recherches anatomiques sur le système tendineux extenseur des doigts de la main. *Annales d'Anatomie Pathologique* (Paris), **14**, 311.

MONTANT, R. & BAUMANN, A. (1938) Rupture luxation de l'appareil extenseur des doigts au niveau de l'art première articulation interphalangienne. *Revue d'Orthopédie*, **25**, 5–22.

MULDER, J. D. & LANDSMEER, J. M. F. (1968) The mechanism of claw finger. *Journal of Bone and Joint Surgery*, **50-B**, 664–668.

MULDER, TH. J. (1970) Röntgen-cinematografie en draadreconstructie van de pols. Thesis: Leiden, Holland.

MUSGRAVE, J. H. (1971) How dextrous was Neanderthal man? *Nature* (London), **233**, 538–541.

MUSGRAVE, J. H. (1972) Some metrical properties of proximal phalanges. *Journal of Anatomy*, **111**, 474–475.

NAPIER, J. R. (1955a) The form and function of the carpo-metacarpal joint of the thumb. *Journal of Anatomy*, **89**, 362–369.

NAPIER, J. R. (1955b) Prehensile movements of the human hand. *Journal of Anatomy*, **89**, 564.

NAPIER, J. R. (1961) Prehensility and opposability in the hands of primates. *Symposium of the Zoological Society of London*, **5**, 115–132.

NAPIER, J. R. (1965) Evolution of the human hand. *Proceedings of the Royal Institution of Great Britain*, **40**, 544–557.

PIERON, A. P. (1973) The mechanism of the first carpometacarpal (CMC) joint. An anatomical and mechanical analysis. *Acta Orthopaedica Scandinavica*, Suppl. 148. Thesis: Leiden, Holland.

RABISCHONG, P. (1962) L'innervation proprioceptive des muscles lombricaux de la main chez l'homme. *Revue de Chirurgie Orthopédique et Réparatrice de l'Appareil Moteur* (Paris), **48**, 234–245.

RICHE. (1897) Le nerf cubital et les muscles de l'éminence thénar. *Bull. et Mém. de la Société Anatomique de Paris*, pp. 251–252.

SALSBURY, C. R. (1937) The interosseous muscles of the hand. *Journal of Anatomy*, **71**, 395–403.

SHREWSBURY, M. M. & KUCZYNSKI, K. (1974) Flexor digitorum superficialis tendon in the fingers of the human hand. *The Hand*, **6**, 121–133.

SHIINO, K. (1925) Einiges über die anatomischen Grundlagen der Greifbewegungen. *Zeitschrift für Anatomie und Entwicklungsgeschichte*, **77**, 344–362.

SMITH, E. M., JUVINALL, R. C., BENDER, L. F. & PEARSON, J. R. (1964) Role of the finger flexors in rheumatoid deformities of the metacarpophalangeal joints. *Arthritis and Rheumatism*, **7**, 467–480.

SMITH, R. D. & MARCARIAN, H. Q. (1966) The muscle spindles of the dorsal and palmar interosseus muscles. *Anatomischer Anzeiger*, **119**, 409–414.

STACK, H. G. (1963) A study of muscle function in the fingers. *Annals of the Royal College of Surgeons of England*, **33**, 307–322.

STACK, H. G. (1973) *The Palmar Fascia*. Edinburgh: Churchill Livingstone.

STILWELL, D. L. (1957) The innervation of deep structures of the hand. *American Journal of Anatomy*, **101**, 75–100.

STOPFORD, J. S. B. (1921) The nerve supply of the interphalangeal and metacarpophalangeal joints. *Journal of Anatomy and Physiology*, **56**, 1–11.

TANDLER, J. (1896) Zur Anatomie der Arterien der Hand. *Anatomische Hefte*, Abt. I, **7**, 263–282.

THOMAS, D. H., LONG, C. & LANDSMEER, J. M. F. (1968) Biomechanical considerations of lumbricalis behaviour in the human finger. *Journal of Biomechanics*, **1**, 107–115.

THOMINE, J. M. (1965) Conjunctif d'enveloppe des doigts et squelette fibreux des commissures interdigitales. *Annales de Chirurgie Plastique*, **10**, 194–203.

TUBIANA, R. & VALENTIN, P. (1963) L'extension des doigts. *Revue de Chirurgie Orthopédique et Réparatrice de l'Appareil Moteur* (Paris), **49**, 543–562.

TUBIANA, R. & VALENTIN, P. (1964) The physiology of the extension of the fingers. *The Surgical Clinics of North America*, **44**, 907–918.

TUTTLE, R. H. (1967) Knuckle-walking and the evolution of hominoid hands. *American Journal of Physical Anthropology*, **26**, 171–206.

TUTTLE, R. H. (1969a) Quantitative and functional studies on the hands of the Anthropoidea. I. The Hominoidea. *Journal of Morphology*, **128**, 309–364.

TUTTLE, R. H. (1969b) Knuckle-walking and the problem of human origins. *Science*, **166**, 953–961.

TUTTLE, R. H., BASMAJIAN, J. V., REGENOS, E. & SHINE, G. (1972) Electromyography of knuckle-walking: results of four experiments on the forearm of Pan Gorilla. *American Journal of Physical Anthropology*, **37**, 255–267.

WEITBRECHT, J. (1742) *Syndesmologia*. Translated by Kaplan, E. B. Philadelphia: Saunders (1969).

WINSLOW, J. B. (1752) *Exposition Anatomique de la Structure du Corps Humain*. 2nd edn., p. 349. Amsterdam.

ZANDER, R. (1890). Über die Nerven des Handrückens und über ihre Bedeutung für die Diagnose von Verletzungen der Armnerven. *Berliner klinische Wochenschrift*, 27. Jhrgang, 172–173.

ZUCKERKANDL, E. (1896) Über die tiefen Hohlhandäste der Arteria Ulnaris. *Anatomische Hefte*, Abt. I, **6**, 533–559.